ASANAS FOR AUTISM AND SPECIAL NEEDS

Jodie,

Thank you for sharing your powerful story! May you continue to shine your beautiful light!

♡ much love,
Shawnee Thornton Hardy

of related interest

Yoga for Children with Autism Spectrum Disorders
A Step-by-Step Guide for Parents and Caregivers
Dion E. Betts and Stacey W. Betts
Foreword by Louise Goldberg and Joshua S. Betts
ISBN 978 1 84310 817 7
eISBN 978 1 84642 498 4

Integrated Yoga
Yoga with a Sensory Integrative Approach
Nicole Cuomo
ISBN 978 1 84310 862 7
eISBN 978 1 84642 677 3

Frog's Breathtaking Speech
How children (and frogs) can use yoga breathing to deal with anxiety, anger and tension
Michael Chissick
Illustrated by Sarah Peacock
ISBN 978 1 84819 091 7
eISBN 978 0 85701 074 2

Ladybird's Remarkable Relaxation
How children (and frogs, dogs, flamingos and dragons) can use yoga relaxation
to help deal with stress, grief, bullying and lack of confidence
Michael Chissick
Illustrated by Sarah Peacock
ISBN 978 1 84819 146 4
eISBN 978 0 85701 112 1

The Autism Fitness Handbook
An Exercise Program to Boost Body Image, Motor Skills, Posture and
Confidence in Children and Teens with Autism Spectrum Disorder
David S. Geslak
Foreword by Stephen M. Shore
ISBN 978 1 84905 998 5
eISBN 978 0 85700 963 0

ASANAS
FOR AUTISM AND SPECIAL NEEDS

Yoga to Help Children with their Emotions,
Self-Regulation and Body Awareness

SHAWNEE THORNTON HARDY

PHOTOGRAPHS BY TIM HARDY

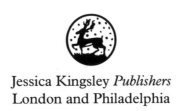

Jessica Kingsley *Publishers*
London and Philadelphia

First published in 2015
by Jessica Kingsley Publishers
73 Collier Street
London N1 9BE, UK
and
400 Market Street, Suite 400
Philadelphia, PA 19106, USA

www.jkp.com

Library of Congress Cataloging in Publication Data
A CIP catalog record for this book is available from the Library of Congress

British Library Cataloguing in Publication Data
A CIP catalogue record for this book is available from the British Library

ISBN 978 1 84905 988 6
eISBN 978 1 78450 059 7

Printed and bound in the United States

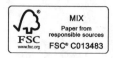

MIX
Paper from
responsible sources
FSC® C013483

I would like to dedicate this book to children with autism and special needs who have taught me to be a better teacher and a better human being, and to the parents, caregivers, teachers and other professionals who dedicate their lives to working with such unique individuals.

Contents

Acknowledgments

I would like to thank Jessica Kingsley Publishers for believing in the value of this topic and helping me share it with the world. I would also like to thank the many professionals, paraprofessionals, parents, guardians and other individuals whom I have worked with throughout the years. Thanks to my mother for instilling a passion for writing and expression early on in my life, to my brothers for showing me that sometimes you just have to go out and create what you want, to my husband for his never-ending support and encouragement, to my daughter Mila for making me strive to be my best every day, to my teachers who have taught me the power of yoga in my own life and most of all to the many children I have worked with throughout the years who have been my inspiration in writing this book.

Disclaimer

Although poses and breathing exercises are taught in a fun and playful way in this book it is important prior to incorporating yoga poses in a child's routine to be aware of any physical limitations, health conditions or challenges the child may have. Many children with special needs may lack a sense of balance, coordination or awareness of their surrounding environment and may have limited fine and gross motor skills. Children with special needs will have a varying degree of flexibility, strength and coordination. It is important to assess the needs of each individual child and make adaptations or modifications in order to support the overall wellbeing and safety of the child when practicing yoga postures. Seated and supine (lying down) yoga postures may be more appropriate for children with poor muscle control or lack of coordination and balance. It is best to start with simpler poses then build up to more challenging poses as the child progresses in their practice. The pictures of poses provided in this book are simply guides and the intention is not that the child looks exactly the same as the photos. Each child will look different in the poses and will require modifications or adjustments based on their unique physical abilities, strengths and challenges. This book is a guide for teaching yoga poses and breathing but it is up to the adult to understand the specific needs of each child prior to introducing them to yoga. Yoga should not replace medical advice or assessment. Specific considerations and precautions must be considered when introducing poses and breathing exercises to a child with special needs.

PREFACE

I look across the room as my students are lying peacefully in their savasana, no sound, and bodies still. I reflect on what a shift this is from their typical display of behaviors such as fidgetiness, stimming, difficulty with focus and at times anxious and disruptive behaviors. I am impressed by the deep and intense focus of the students during the practice of asanas (physical postures) and how they have become so much more aware of their bodies and where they are in space. I draw upon the moment when a class was beginning and the students were droopy eyed and lacked the energy to focus and one of my student's raised her hand and said, "Ms. Thornton, I think we should do bee breath so we can be more awake and pay attention." I remember a time when I asked a student how dragon's breath made her feel and she said, "It helps me get out my anger." I remember when one of my students approached me after yoga and said, "Ms. Thornton, thank you for helping me find my Qi." I think of the many drawings a student has given me of he and his friends on their yoga mats "doing yoga." I remember my conversations with parents telling me their child is doing yoga poses at home that they have learned at school. I smile inside thinking about morning group and how every day the students draw their palms together to their foreheads and I say to the students, "When we say Namaste, what are we sharing?" and they say "Our light."

I write this preface with great enthusiasm and passion. Over the years I have worked with hundreds of children with special needs with a variety of challenges, personalities, characteristics and abilities. What I have found to be a common thread amongst most of the children I have worked with is their struggle coping with anxiety, expressing their emotions and self-regulating their emotional and physical states. I have witnessed the impact anxiety and the lack of communication and coping skills have had on these children. They struggle with developing and maintaining social relationships and being part of the world around them.

They struggle with communicating their wants and needs and feelings towards others. They struggle with health problems such as weak immune systems, digestive disorders, insomnia and autoimmune related problems. Many children I have worked with over the years have made huge gains with communication, self-regulation, behavior and academic skills when provided with positive behavior supports, sensory integration supports, visual aids for communication and understanding and a kinesthetic and individualized approach to learning. It wasn't until I began to immerse myself in learning the therapeutics of yoga that I realized what was missing from their programing in the home and school setting. Through my studies I have learned the devastating impact stress and anxiety can have on our overall health and wellbeing. I now see how everything is interconnected and I have a greater understanding of the autonomic nervous system, how our response to stress can affect our bodies, mood, behavior, thinking and ability to learn. When we are over-stressed, everything is impacted: language and communication, cognition, relationships with others and optimal functioning of our body. I have come to the enlightened understanding that we need to look at these children from a "holistic" perspective. My goal in writing this book is to teach children with special needs *mindfulness* of their own bodies, thoughts and behaviors. My goal is to teach children with special needs how to *breathe* and *move their bodies* so they may learn to calm their nervous systems and change their stress responses in order to live happier, calmer and healthier lives.

Children with autism and many other special needs can struggle with heightened levels of anxiety, over-stimulation, difficulty communicating, limited body awareness and a variety of physical and sensory needs. Yoga for children with autism and special needs can provide a variety of benefits, such as learning skills of relaxation and focus and developing coping mechanisms for anxiety and stress. The combination of asanas (postures), pranayama (breath work) and deep relaxation will strengthen the child's nervous system, increase overall health and facilitate the development of body awareness and concentration. By integrating yoga into their lives, children with autism and special needs can gain new motor, communication and social skills as well as body and breath awareness, self-regulation skills and increased self-confidence and self-esteem. The end result is an overall improvement in their quality of life.

Children with autism and many children with special needs will often have difficulty with expressive and receptive language. Specific teaching strategies must be used to keep the child engaged and support understanding. Often children with communication and language difficulties will exhibit negative or disruptive behaviors as an attempt to communicate wants, needs or feelings.

Many children with language processing delays, unique sensory needs and/or communication difficulties can experience high levels of anxiety, over-stimulation or under-stimulation. The incorporation of yoga at home or in the classroom teaches children to be aware of their physical and emotional states. This book will support children's language processing delays and difficulty with communication by providing suggestions of visual tools necessary for learning, retaining and incorporating the skills into their daily lives.

Managing the challenges of a child with special needs can be stressful, difficult and often overwhelming for parents, caregivers, teachers and the child. I have worked with many families and caregivers throughout the years, consulting and helping develop positive behavior programs, visual strategies and communication tools to support the child and family's needs within the school and home setting. The practice of yoga as a family unit can not only be healing for the family but it can also be a fun and exciting way to spend time together, bond, develop better communication and create a calm and peaceful home environment. This book can be a tool for parents, caregivers, educators and other professionals who work in the field of special education to support and teach:

▶ self-regulation and self-soothing of physical and emotional states

▶ body awareness

▶ awareness of breath

▶ balance

▶ hand–eye coordination

▶ focus

▶ coping strategies

▶ language and communication

▶ strength and flexibility

▶ self-confidence

▶ motor skills

▶ social skills.

This book will give parents, teachers, caregivers and educators the tools to teach simple yoga poses and breathing exercises to children with autism and special needs in a step-by-step manner. The pictures and language are simplified so the child can connect and learn. Poses and breathing can be taught in a repetitious manner with consistent language for optimal learning and understanding.

I have seen the benefits of yoga for children with special needs first hand through incorporating yoga into my classroom and teaching yoga through individual sessions to children with special needs. Their response has been so positive that it has inspired me to write this book. My hope is that this book will be the beginning to a lifelong love and practice of yoga for children with special needs. My desire is that through the practice of yoga poses and mindful breathing, these beautiful individuals will experience life with less anxiety and more balance so they may shine their lights with brightness and magnificence for all to see.

1

WHAT IS YOGA?

A simplified definition of yoga is union or to "yoke" which refers to a unification of the mind, body and spirit. A more contemporary outlook towards yoga is that the practice of yoga allows for cessation or stilling of the mind, which in turn relaxes the body. Yoga originated over 10,000 years ago in India. In the last decade, yoga has become a popular practice in the west. Although yoga has many different lineages and styles, it has recently become known for its many benefits to physical and emotional health and wellbeing. Yoga is thought to minimize the impact of stress on the individual. Yogic science believes that the regular practice of pranayama and asanas strengthens the nervous system and helps people face stressful situations and events more positively (Iyengar 2008). The two key components that are universal to the practice of yoga are pranayama (breath) and asana (poses). Various forms of meditation, visualization practices and guided imagery are also incorporated in the practice of yoga.

Pranayama, in simple terms, is the practice of breathing techniques that help with calming and/or energizing the mind and body. Many children with autism and other special needs who experience high levels of anxiety and difficulty coping with stress struggle with mindful breathing. Often times when they are anxious and their bodies respond in a fight/flight mode they will either hold their breath (not breathe) or breathe rapidly. Children can learn fun and interactive breathing techniques that will help them cope with stress, anxiety and difficult emotions and will calm their nervous systems in order to bring their bodies to a more regulated state.

Asanas are based on three basic human postures of standing, sitting or lying down. The practice of asana has a beneficial impact on the whole body. Asanas tone the muscles, and strengthen tendons and ligaments. Asanas also strengthen the nervous, lymphatic and metabolic systems. Asanas can be adapted or modified to meet the needs of any physical or development ability. Through asana practice one develops increased balance, strength and flexibility. Asanas also relax the mind and body, which allows the body to recover from stress and fatigue, strengthening the immune system. Certain asanas are considered to be very beneficial for digestive health, which can be an area in which children with autism and special needs are affected, due to stress, anxiety and limited diet preferences. The practice of asanas (poses) for kids with autism and special needs supports them in learning body parts, understanding where their bodies are in space (body awareness) and increases concentration, focus, flexibility, strength, balance, self-regulation and self-confidence/self-esteem.

Meditation and visualizations are used in the practice of yoga to bring focus and calming to the mind. There can be many forms of meditation. Visualization strategies such as envisioning a relaxing image or envisioning a soothing color can be ways in which one focuses and calms the mind, in turn bringing a calmer state to the body. The use of visualization strategies and guided imagery for children with special needs supports them with calming the mind and body, concentration, language development and imagination.

WHAT DOES NAMASTE MEAN?

At the end of many yoga practices, the teacher will bring their palms together with thumbs touching their forehead and will bow to their students while saying "Namaste," then bringing their palms to their heart center or heart chakra. Traditionally, Namaste signifies the unity or connection of the teacher and the students. It is an offering of gratitude from the teacher to the students and the students to the teacher for sharing knowledge, space, energy and their hearts with one another. When I say Namaste with the children I explain to them that when we say Namaste we are sharing our lights, what is special and unique about us as individuals. It is an opportunity to celebrate and embrace our unique differences and abilities and share them with one another. It is also my genuine offering of gratitude from myself to the children for being teachers in my life and sharing their lights with me. Namaste is also a signal or cue that the practice is complete or has come to an end. It is up to the adult whether they prefer to teach Namaste to the child at the end of the practice. It is a common gesture in the practice of yoga but is not a necessary element to a child's practice.

WHAT IS SANSKRIT?

Sanskrit is a classical literary language of India. Most traditional poses practiced in the west have now been given English terms; however, most of the traditional yoga poses have Sanskrit names. I have included the Sanskrit names for poses in this book as a reference for the adult. There are many resources available throughout the web on the subject of yoga. Having the Sanskrit names of poses can be helpful when looking up information. I find that many of the children I teach enjoy practicing the Sanskrit words for poses. They get excited about learning to say poses in another language. However, the words in Sanskrit can be long and may be difficult for the children to pronounce. I teach the children Sanskrit words by clapping with the syllables (example—suk-ha-sa-na for sukhasana; Sanskrit for easy pose or cross-legged pose). Many of the poses in this book have made-up English names to suit the interests of children. It is up to the adult to know the children's language abilities in order to decide whether they should teach the Sanskrit names of poses along with English.

WHAT IS DRISHTI?

Drishti is a specific focal point where the gaze rests during asanas and meditation. Drishti encourages focus, concentration and helps with balance. Drishti allows the mind to focus on one focal point so it does not wander. Focusing on one point also encourages relaxation and being in the present moment.

2

YOGA FOR AUTISM
AND SPECIAL NEEDS

In order to understand the benefits of yoga for children with special needs, it is important to understand the characteristics and challenges that come with each disability. The practice of yoga can be beneficial for any individual or child but can be particularly supportive to children with special needs due to their many physical, physiological and emotional difficulties. The specific disabilities identified in this book include ASD (autism spectrum disorder), ADD/ADHD (attention deficit disorder or attention deficit hyperactive disorder), Fragile X, Down syndrome and Prader Willi. Although these specific disabilities are identified, the poses, breaths and strategies suggested would be appropriate for a variety of disabilities, including, but not limited to, children with developmental delays, anxiety disorders, ED (emotionally disturbed), OHI (other health impairment) and cerebral palsy. The poses and approach to teaching yoga can be modified to meet the needs of low functioning as well as high functioning children with special needs.

Autism is a group of developmental brain disorders, collectively called ASD (autism spectrum disorder). The term "spectrum" refers to the wide range of skills, levels of impairment, functioning, symptoms and disability. A child with ASD may present from mild impairment to severely disabled. The DSM-5™ (Desk Reference to the Diagnostic Criteria from DSM–5) specifies the diagnostic criteria for ASD as having persistent deficits in social interaction across multiple contexts (APA 2013) in conjunction with restrictive or repetitive patterns of behavior. The spectrum of disorders identified as ASD include:

- autistic disorder (classic autism)
- Asperger's disorder (Asperger syndrome)
- pervasive developmental disorder not otherwise specified (PDD-NOS)
- Rett's disorder (Rett syndrome)
- childhood disintegrative disorder (CDD).

According to the *Desk Reference to the Diagnostic Criteria from DSM-5* (APA 2013*)*, Children with ASD exhibit deficits in social–emotional reciprocity such as having a reciprocal conversation, responding to or initiating social interactions, sharing or understanding emotions, affect and interests of others. Children with ASD also exhibit deficits in non-verbal as well as verbal communication. Some children have relatively normal communication, some have limited language and some may not use spoken language at all. Children with ASD may have difficulty with eye contact, understanding and using gestures, body language or context cues in social interactions and communication. Children with ASD vary widely in intelligence, abilities and behaviors. Restrictive or repetitive patterns of behavior, interests or activities are also evident. Some typical behaviors include stereotypes of repetitive motor movement with the use of objects or with speech, such as repetitively lining items up in an organized pattern or using echolalia (repetition of words or phrases the child has heard). Unusual responses to sensory information such as bright lights, loud noises and temperature may also be present. According to the National Institute of Child Health and Human Development, children with ASD may also develop co-occurring mental disorders including ADHD, anxiety or depression (NICHD 2013). Many children with ASD may also develop OCD (obsessive compulsive disorder).

The National Institute of Child Health and Human Development (NICHD 2013) explains that the main signs and symptoms of ASD involve problems in the following areas:

- difficulty using and understanding language (expressive and receptive language)
- difficulty relating to people, objects and events; for example, lack of eye contact, pointing behavior and lack of facial responses; limited social skills and social awareness
- unusual play or fixation with toys and other objects
- difficulty with changes in routine or familiar surroundings

- ▶ repetitive body movements or behavior patterns, such as hand flapping, hair twirling, foot tapping, or more complex movements

- ▶ inability to cuddle or be comforted

- ▶ difficulty regulating behaviors and emotions, which may result in temper tantrums, anxiety and aggression.

Children with ASD struggle across all environments with language, communication, social skills, sensory issues, body awareness, handling change in routine or environment, awareness of their and others' emotions, anxiety and many other issues. Explicit teaching of social skills, language, emotional regulation and body awareness are necessary for children with ASD. Due to the many challenges children with ASD face, they may exhibit behaviors deemed as negative or socially inappropriate. Although there are many theories, the exact cause of ASD is not clear.

ADD/ADHD

Attention deficit hyperactivity disorder (ADHD) is a disorder that appears in early childhood. It can be referred to as attention deficit disorder or ADD as well as attention deficit hyperactivity disorder or ADHD. According to the *Desk Reference to the Diagnostic Criteria from DSM-5*, ADHD involves "a persistent pattern of inattention and/or hyperactivity—impulsivity that interferes with functioning or development" (APA 2013, p.31). Children with ADD/ADHD can have difficulty inhibiting their spontaneous responses—responses that can involve everything from movement, social situations, speech and attentiveness. Although multiple factors have been indicated, the exact cause of ADD/ADHD is not yet clear.

The most common features of ADD/ADHD include:

- ▶ difficulty sustaining attention (inattention)

- ▶ impulsive behaviors (impulsivity)

- ▶ hyperactive behavior (hyperactivity).

A child with ADD/ADHD may struggle with paying attention in school, as well as other activities that require focus, can be forgetful, may have difficulty organizing thoughts and completing tasks or projects and may have difficulty with listening skills and following directions. Children who have the *hyperactive* component of ADHD may have difficulty staying still, may bounce from one task to the next, may talk excessively or have difficulty waiting for their turn to speak. Many children with ADHD can be very impulsive both socially and emotionally and may have a quick temper or "short fuse." A child with ADHD can often be described as "their motor is constantly running." They often struggle with self-calming and self-regulation of their physical and emotional states. These factors can greatly affect the child's interactions with others and their ability to make friends and maintain friendships. Some children with ADD/ADHD may hyper-focus on a specific task or activity and may have difficulty when asked to switch to a new task or activity. Due to difficulty with focus, children with ADHD may struggle with following directions or attending to verbal language. Many children with ADD/ADHD may also present as having difficulties with sensory integration and sensory processing.

FRAGILE X

According to the National Institute of Child Health and Human Development (NICHD 2013), Fragile X syndrome (FXS) is a genetic disorder. It results in a wide range of developmental, physical and behavioral problems and is the most common known cause of inherited developmental disability worldwide. Twice as many males than females inherit Fragile X.

Common features of Fragile X include:

▶ attention deficit disorders with or without hyperactivity

▶ anxiety (hyper-arousal)

▶ extreme reaction or aversion to sensory stimuli (loud noise, touch, strong smells or tastes, eye contact), SPD—sensory processing disorder

▶ difficulties with expressive and receptive language

▶ sleep difficulties

▶ autism-like features including hand flapping and biting (or chewing on clothes)

▶ poor eye contact and resistance to changes in routine.

Due to their heightened sensitivity to sensory stimuli, difficulty with communication and high levels of anxiety many children with Fragile X may exhibit unusual or challenging behaviors. Children with Fragile X can present with mild to moderate or severe cognitive impairment. It is common for children with Fragile X to exhibit obsessive-compulsive or repetitive behaviors or become fixated on thoughts, ideas or specific objects. Children with Fragile X share many common features with those with ASD and often benefit from similar strategies and supports in the home and school setting as children with ASD. Around one in three children who have Fragile X syndrome also meet the diagnostic criteria for ASD (NICHD 2006).

DOWN SYNDROME

According to the National Down Syndrome Society (NDSS 2014), Down syndrome is the most common and readily identifiable chromosomal condition associated with intellectual disabilities. It is caused by a chromosomal abnormality. In most cases, the diagnosis of Down syndrome is made according to results from a chromosome test administered shortly after birth. There is a wide variation in mental abilities, behavior and developmental progress in individuals with Down syndrome. Their level of intellectual disability may range from mild to severe, with the majority functioning in the mild to moderate range.

Common features of Down syndrome include:

▶ language processing disorders (receptive and expressive language)

▶ cognitive delays

▶ short attention span

▶ impulsive behavior

▶ anxiety or depression

▶ hyper-flexibility (excessive ability to extend the joints)

▶ poor muscle tone

▶ thyroid conditions, more often low thyroid

▶ digestive problems

▶ sleep difficulties

▶ delays in fine and gross motor development

▶ hearing and vision disorders

▶ sensory integration dysfunction.

Children with Down syndrome who have difficulty with expressive or receptive language may exhibit behaviors due to frustration with communication. Many children with Down syndrome may have co-occurring anxiety disorders, ADHD or attention problems as well as sensory integration difficulties, which can affect their behavior as well as socialization and participation in activities. Some children with Down syndrome may also have a co-occurring diagnosis of autism (approximately 5–7%). Obsessive-compulsive behaviors and fixation on specific objects or thoughts may also be present (NDSS 2014).

PRADER WILLI

According to the Genetics Home Reference (GHR 2014), Prader Willi is a genetic disorder that affects 1 in 10,000–30,000 individuals worldwide. Many individuals with Prader Willi may have common physical characteristics such as short stature, small hands and feet and puberty is often delayed or incomplete. Beginning in childhood, affected individuals develop an insatiable appetite (hyperphagia), which leads to chronic overeating and often obesity. Many children with Prader Willi develop an obsession with food which can affect their home life as well as their ability to participate in social events or activities with others. Individuals with Prader Willi frequently have mild to moderate intellectual impairment and cognitive disabilities.

Common features of Prader Willi are:

▶ poor muscle tone

▶ behavioral issues

▶ difficulty regulating emotions

▶ compulsive behaviors (picking at skin)

▶ obsessive behaviors

▶ difficulty with communication

▶ sensory integration dysfunction (sensory processing disorder)

▶ delayed fine and gross motor skills

▶ anxiety.

Due to their extreme obsession with food, children with Prader Willi can experience high levels of anxiety along with obsessive-compulsive behaviors. They often display immature social behavior and may lack understanding of personal boundaries or space towards others. Part of the reason for their lack of awareness of personal space is their difficulty with body awareness (where their bodies are in relationship to others). They may present with difficulties in communicating their emotions, self-regulation and coping skills. Children with Prader Willi may display inappropriate behaviors due to the many challenges of their disability. It is common for children with Prader Willi to have underactive thyroids, which affects their metabolism, level of energy and overall health.

Children with autism spectrum disorder, Fragile X, Prader Willi, Down syndrome and ADD/ADHD share many common factors with their disabilities as well as similar responses to stress. The most common features include anxiety, difficulty with communication, difficulty self-regulating physical and emotional states and with body awareness and sleep difficulties. Many children identified with these disabilities exhibit obsessive-compulsive or repetitive behaviors. These children have the same feelings and emotions as anyone else. Stress, anxiety, worry, fear and anger, are all typical feelings that children have. Often children with ASD and other special needs do not know how to communicate their feelings or emotions and will exhibit their response to stress in inappropriate manners. These children have more difficulty with emotional regulation, making it more challenging for them to identify levels of emotions and regulate their intensity. In addition, many children with special needs have more trigger points that cause heightened anxiety.

There is sufficient evidence that children with autism are more likely to suffer from high levels of anxiety as compared to their neuro-typical peers. One study done to report on the prevalence of anxiety and mood problems among 9 to 14-year-old children with Asperger syndrome (AS) and high functioning autism found that compared with a sample of 1751 community children AS and autistic children demonstrated a greater rate of anxiety and depression problems. These problems had a significant impact on their overall adaptation (Kim *et al.* 2000). According to the *International Journal of Yoga Therapy*, yoga therapeutic interventions have been successful in addressing each one of the core symptoms associated with autism spectrum disorder (Ehleringer 2010).

While the academic research on the use of yoga for children is more limited than that of adults and is even more limited for that of children with special needs, what has been done suggests that children improve their grades, behavior in school, physical health and attitudes towards themselves. In "Teaching Yoga in Urban elementary schools", Harper suggests that yoga-based activities have the potential to reduce stress and anxiety, increase health and wellness and teach emotional regulation (2010).

One study tested the effects of yoga on adolescents with anxiety, depression and medical illness. The participants consisted of 21 adolescents aged 13–18 years who obtained a clinically significant score on the anxiety, depression or somatization subscales of the Behavior Assessment Scale for Children (BASC).

The adolescents participated in 150-minute classes one time per week and were encouraged to practice at home with two yoga DVDs. The final results of the study concluded that the eight week yoga intervention positively impacted targeted symptoms of stress and physical fitness for the adolescents who completed the eight weeks (Kaley-Isley *et al.* 2009).

An additional study was done to evaluate the potential benefits of yoga for adolescent musicians. The adolescent music students were aged 13–18 and were enrolled in a prestigious summer music program that was thought to be a high stress/high pressure program. The music students participated in a six-week yoga research program at the Kripalu Yoga Center. The total group consisted of 84 participants, 51 being in the control group. The participants attended three yoga classes per week and completed self-report questionnaires at baseline and at the end of the program for performance anxiety, positive psychological characteristics, mindfulness, mood and perceived benefit of yoga. The results of the study revealed significant improvements in the participants' moods, levels of stress, anxiety and ability to cope with stress in their program and overall mental clarity and mindfulness (Shorter *et al.* 2008).

While these studies suggest the practice of yoga helps adolescents with stress, anxiety, coping skills, mood and mindfulness, additional studies have been done to identify the effects of yoga practice as an intervention in the classroom or school setting. Schools are increasingly using yoga therapy to help manage stress and influence wellbeing and behavior. The increased awareness of the potential benefits of yoga for children has resulted in school programs that address anxiety and stress by treating the body and mind. Yoga in the school setting has been reported as calming children, reducing obesity, reducing discipline problems, decreasing anger and panic attacks and enhancing imagination, concentration and academic performance (Flisek 2001). A review of articles of yoga for school-age children revealed a variety of outcomes. Evidence suggests that yoga is associated with improved cardiovascular status, physical functioning and behavior (Galantino, Galbavy and Quinn 2008).

According to Jensen and Kenny (2004), yoga may improve attention and emotional control. Jensen and Kenny studied 19 boys who had been clinically diagnosed with ADHD and randomly assigned them to either a yoga treatment group or a cooperative activities group. Although both groups of boys showed improvement in certain measured behaviors, the yoga group had more favorable changes in factors such as emotional liability, restlessness and impulsive behavior. Subjects who participated in additional home practice of yoga showed an even greater response (Jensen and Kenny 2004).

Whether yoga is done with adults or adolescents, there are numerous studies on the effects of yoga on the brain and levels of anxiety. A study published in *The Journal of Alternative and Complementary Medicine* found that certain types of yoga sessions (a focus on yoga posture, as opposed to breathing) increase gamma-aminobutyric acid (GABA) levels in the brain. Anxiety is associated with low GABA levels. GABA is the primary neurotransmitter known to counterbalance the excitatory neurotransmitter glutamate, which in the case of anxiety is over-active. The study found that yoga participants had greater reductions in anxiety and greater improvements in mood than people who walked for exercise. These mood improvements and reductions in anxiety were correlated to changes in GABA levels. The increase of activity in the GABA system found the effects of using yoga postures are similar to the effects of medications prescribed for anxiety (Streeter *et al.* 2007).

Many children with autism and other special needs may struggle with coping in their day-to-day lives in both the home and school setting. The combination of high levels of anxiety, lack of coping and communication skills and difficulty with self-regulation can result in children "acting out," having difficulty staying engaged in a task and participating in life activities with their families, peers and other individuals. The practice of yoga, incorporating asana (postures) and pranayama (breath) can be a tremendous tool in helping children with autism and other special needs cope with their anxiety, manage their stress and respond to sensory stimuli in a more positive manner. When a child with special needs feels heightened levels of stress or anxiety, their sympathetic nervous system responds in a fight or flight mode. The sympathetic nervous system responds by increasing the heart rate, speeding up breathing, sending out stress hormones to the body and essentially shutting down the cognitive or "thinking" part of the brain. Yoga can allow the child to tap into the parasympathetic nervous system or the "resting system" in order to bring their bodies and minds to a calmer state. Lack of sleep or abnormal sleep patterns can be a major factor in a child's ability to focus, complete daily activities and cope with stress. Many children with special needs exhibit irregular sleep problems or insomnia. Insomnia or lack of enough sleep can increase chances of experiencing symptoms of anxiety or depression, weakens the immune system, decreases the ability to focus and concentrate, slows the digestive process and affects ability to regulate emotional responses to stress. Yoga supports healthy sleep patterns by bringing the body and mind to a calmer state. Specific poses can be practiced prior to bedtime to decrease insomnia. Getting more rest can have a significant impact on a child's health, communication and expression of emotions, coping skills and overall wellness.

TEACHING YOGA TO CHILDREN WITH AUTISM AND SPECIAL NEEDS

Because of the unique challenges children with autism and other special needs face, specific strategies must be used to teach yoga. It is important to note that each individual child will require a different level of support or modification. Some children with a higher level of language development and physical ability may be more capable of following verbal cues and doing poses with minimal modifications, other children may require more modeling, physical prompting and modification to poses. The key to introducing yoga to a child with special needs is to make it fun, interactive and to teach poses that allow them to feel successful. As the child learns poses and breathing strategies through repetition, new and more challenging poses can be introduced to build self-esteem and self-confidence.

Visuals, visuals, visuals

Many children with autism and other special needs may struggle with processing verbal language. Because they struggle with receptive language, they often respond more positively to visual supports that aid in understanding and retaining information. Visual supports help children with language processing deficits transition more smoothly to activities, relieves the stress and anxiety of having to remember what comes next and supports memory, word retrieval, language and communication. Visual supports can make learning more interesting and interactive, which in turn becomes more motivating to the child. Use as many visuals as possible. Children with language deficits respond far better to visual cues than they do verbal cues. Verbal cues can easily be lost and misunderstood due to deficits in receptive language (how they receive and process verbal language). A majority of the poses and breathing strategies taught in this book are named after an animal or object and can be represented in a variety of visual ways. This is a benefit because many children with disabilities identified in this book, particularly autism, often find it easier to relate to objects than people.

Modeling

Modeling the pose yourself to the child will support them in learning the poses. It will always be a benefit to model the pose and breath to the child while using verbal and visual cues.

Using images and pictures

Printing out or drawing pictures of the animals, landscapes or other objects that go with the pose or breath may help motivate the child and keep them interested and engaged. The child will be more likely to retain the information and memory of the pose if there is a visual connected to it. Simple drawings of stick figures in the pose will help the child process what the pose looks like so they can explore the pose in their own bodies.

Pictures of the child doing the pose or breath

Many children with special needs may have difficulty relating to others. They can often be self-focused and may have little interest in those around them. Taking pictures of the child doing the pose can be an easier way for them to connect to the pose and see the relationship of the pose to themselves and their own body.

Word and picture walls

Displaying pictures of the pose or breath with the word next to the picture will give the child daily exposure to the poses and breath and will help the child learn and retain the information and vocabulary in their memory banks. Matching pictures to words supports language, vocabulary development and communication.

Social stories

Many children with language deficits respond well to social stories because they are able to process the information more easily when it is presented through words and pictures. Social stories can be created when first introducing yoga to a child with special needs. Social stories can be used to teach a child a single pose, breath or a sequence of poses.

Rule of Five

When it is necessary to use verbal language, follow the Rule of Five. Try not to use more than five words when speaking to the child, speak slowly and clearly and use very specific and concrete language. Every child with special needs will present with varying levels of language processing skills. Adjusting the amount of verbal cues to fit the needs of the child will support the child in processing information and will reduce frustration.

Create a schedule or routine

Often children with autism and other special needs develop a sense of rigidity or need for repetition and sameness. The practice of yoga breath and poses can complement this need as children can learn sequences of poses and breathing through repetition and practice. Developing a schedule or routine of poses will allow the child to feel a sense of control and awareness of what to expect. Allowing the child to choose poses for the sequence will assist them in feeling a sense of importance and involvement in their yoga practice. Having the ability to make choices allows the child to feel more in control over their environment. Using laminated images or actual photographs of the child or someone else in the pose with velcro on the back can allow for the poses to be interchangeable in order for the child or adult to create a variety of sequences on a schedule.

Augmentative communication devices and technology

Children with language processing deficits may have access to an augmentative communication device as a communication tool to support them with receptive and expressive language. There are various forms of augmentative communication devices from a PEC (Picture Exchange Communication) board to a higher level of augmentative device such as a computer. A common device that is being used as a tool for language and communication is the iPad. Specific apps can be utilized to create social stories about yoga poses and breaths as well as schedules and routines for a yoga practice. The camera and video on the iPad allows the adult to take pictures and videos of the child and upload them to various apps on the device. The child can have access to social stories and visuals during times away from their yoga practice to support retention and memory of poses and breaths. It can also be used as a tool for video modeling.

Video modeling

Video modeling is a mode of teaching that uses video recordings to provide a visual model of a targeted behavior or skill. Videotaping the child doing poses and breathing strategies or videotaping other children or adults demonstrating the poses/breaths, then allowing the child to practice along while watching the video, can be motivating, interactive, engaging and will also allow them to see and model the physical movement, sound or action of each pose or breath. An example of a video model would be videotaping a sequence of an adult or another child exhibiting an emotion such as anger or frustration, the adult or another child doing the breath to release that emotion and the adult or another child exhibiting a calm/relaxed feeling after doing the breath. The adult can also videotape the child with special needs moving through the sequence. Video modeling will support the child in developing imitation skills, following multi-step motor activities, learning poses and breathing strategies independently and learning information through repetition. The great thing about video modeling is it is consistent, can be viewed anytime, anywhere and can be watched as many times as necessary for the child to learn the skills taught in the video.

The more visual support, modeling, repetition and exposure to language and vocabulary, the more likely the child will respond to practicing yoga. The key to introducing yoga to a child with special needs is to use as many tools possible to set the child up for success. Along with increased self-confidence and self-esteem, the child will develop increased language and communication skills, self-regulation skills, increased body awareness and hopefully a lifelong connection to yoga.

Positive reinforcement

Using positive reinforcement such as verbal praise, stickers and rewards following completion of a pose, breath or sequence of poses and breathing can help in motivating the child to learn and practice yoga.

3

TEACHING BODY PARTS

Children with ASD and other special needs often have difficulty identifying even the simplest parts of their bodies. Teaching body parts as a preparation for teaching asanas (poses) will support the child in knowing what body parts to move and hold during their yoga practice. Many children with special needs struggle with directional concepts such as left and right or top and bottom. Integrating specific "teaching" of body parts and directional concepts will help the child develop increased body awareness as well as an increased mind–body or brain–body connection. Body parts and directional concepts can be taught in fun and interactive ways to increase motivation as well as retention of learned concepts.

A selection of activities for teaching body parts follows.

AUDITORY AND KINESTHETIC

Many children with special needs respond positively to music and singing. Children also respond well to moving their bodies to music. The repetition of movement and song together will assist the child in retaining information and learning body parts in a fun and exciting way. This specific song will teach the child many of the body parts that are most often emphasized in yoga poses.

SING SONG *HEAD, NECK, SHOULDERS, WRISTS AND ELBOWS*
Concepts learned

▷ rhythm

▷ body parts

▷ body awareness

▷ vocabulary

Instructions for activity

(Sing song to the melody of *Head, Shoulders, Knees and Toes.*)

As you lead the child through the song, have the child touch the parts of the body correlating with the song (adult is modeling the whole time). Have the child sing along if they are verbal and know the song or just have the child touch the body parts with you as you sing. Repeat the song at least three times and practice often!

Head, neck, shoulders, wrists and elbows
Hips and knees and ankles and toes
Head, neck, shoulders wrists and elbows!

Additional suggestion

Videotape yourself or the child singing and modeling the *Head, Neck, Shoulders, Wrists and Elbows* song so they have a visual video model available and can watch the video before they practice their yoga poses as a review or front-loading of body parts.

TAP TAP TAP YOUR BODY PARTS
Concepts learned

▷ body parts

▷ body awareness

▷ rhythm

▷ vocabulary

▷ top to bottom

Instructions for activity

In this activity the child will learn body parts by tapping them repetitively to music. The repetition of language along with movement will support the child in developing memory connections with vocabulary words to body parts. Have child choose a favorite song or adult can choose a song. Begin with top of head and work your way down. Adult can model tapping body parts and vocabulary to the child. Adult says tap your head three times while tapping top of head and saying "Head, head, head." Repeat for all body parts.

Sequence of body parts

Head, neck, shoulders, elbows, wrists, palms, fingers, belly, spine, bottom, hips, knees, ankles, heels, toes.

TACTILE AND KINESTHETIC

Children love learning through tactile and kinesthetic activities. Many children with language processing deficits are tactile learners, meaning they learn best through hands on and movement activities which involve multiple senses. Integrating tactile and kinesthetic activities can be motivating to the child and also increases their understanding and retention of information.

TRACE AND LABEL MY BODY

Concepts learned

▷ body parts

▷ vocabulary

▷ body awareness

You will need

▷ roll of butcher paper

▷ marker (any color)

▷ labels of body parts (suggestion: include picture of body part on label)

Instructions for activity

Have the child lie down on the butcher paper. Trace the child's body. Allow the child to draw a face on the body. Tell the child "We are going to label your body parts." Start with the head and move down. As you label the parts of the body, have the child touch the part on their own body. If the child is capable of writing the body part allow them to label the parts by writing the names of the parts on the body.

Body parts

Head, neck, shoulders, wrists, fingers, belly, hips, knees, ankles, toes.

Put the poster up in the child's room or space where they practice yoga as a visual tool to refer to during yoga practice. Review the poster with the child often or as desired.

USING GAMES

Using games to teach body parts and vocabulary is a fun and interactive way to get the child interested and engaged in learning. Game time with the family provides an opportunity for the family to have fun interacting together, supports socialization and communication and helps the child and family members develop healthy relationships with one another.

GO FISH

This game requires at least two players.

What does the child learn?

▷ communication skills

▷ vocabulary

▷ turn-taking

▷ counting

▷ good sportsmanship

▷ body parts

▷ body awareness

Materials

▷ Pairs of yoga cards with matching body parts (these cards can be printed photos/images of the child's body parts or someone else's body parts). Body parts to include: head, neck, shoulder, arm, elbow, wrist, palm, fingers, chest, belly, hips, bottom, spine/back, knee, ankle, heel, foot, toes.

▷ Visual cue (if needed): Go Fish and Do you have_____? (Adult can write "Go Fish and Do you have _____?" on a whiteboard or piece of paper or enter the cues into the child's communication device so the child has access to the verbal scripts throughout the game.)

How to play the game

1. The adult passes 5–7 cards out to the child and the other player/players and places spare cards in a pile.

2. Each player checks to see if they have matching body parts.

3. Players set pairs aside.

4. One player asks for example: "Do you have elbow?" and touches his/her own elbow.

5. If the other player has the matching pose, they give the card to asking player.

6. If the other player does not have the matching card, they say "Go Fish."

7. The asking player takes a card from the pile.

8. If the player gets a match from the pile, player sets pair aside.

9. Players take turns.

10. The game is over when one person has no more cards in their hand.

11. The person with no cards left in their hand is the winner!

BODY PART MEMORY GAME

This game can be played with one or more players.

What does the child learn?

▷ communication

▷ vocabulary

▷ memory skills

▷ turn-taking

▷ counting

▷ body parts

▷ body awareness

▷ good sportsmanship

Materials

▷ Pairs of matching yoga cards with body parts (these cards can be printed photos/images of the child's body parts or someone else's body parts). Body parts to include: head, neck, shoulder, arm, elbow, wrist, palm, fingers, chest, belly, hips, bottom, spine/back, knee, ankle, heel, foot, toes.

How to play the game

1. Lay all cards face down on a table.

2. Player chooses a card.

3. Player chooses another card.

4. If the cards don't match the player puts the cards back in their spots and the next player goes.

5. If the cards match the player puts the matching set aside and takes another turn. Player keeps going as long as player gets a match.

6. When all of the cards have been matched, players count their cards.

7. The one with the most cards is the winner!

BODY BINGO

This game can be played with one or more players.

What does the child learn?

▷ memory skills

▷ vocabulary

▷ body parts

▷ picture discrimination

▷ turn-taking

▷ visual and listening skills

▷ communication

Materials

▷ Bingo cards with body parts made on the computer or from pictures pasted on paper (each Bingo card has different body parts or body parts arranged in different places). Suggested body parts: head, neck, shoulder, arm, wrist, fingers, chest, belly, spine, hips, knee, ankle, heel, foot, toes).

▷ Pictures of body parts to match pictures on Bingo cards.

▷ Bingo counters (any objects that could be used to place on Bingo spots).

▷ "Bingo" cue or script (in device, written on paper or on a PEC).

How to play the game

1. Each player gets a Bingo card with pictures of body parts.

2. Adult or guide holds up a picture of a body part.

3. The adult or guide can say the name of the body part or ask the child to identify the body part verbally or by pointing to the body part on their body.

4. Players who have the body part on their Bingo card put a marker on the spot.

5. Repeat until a player fills up a row or all of the squares on their Bingo card.

6. Player says "Bingo" if their row is full or their Bingo card is full.

7. The first player to say "Bingo" correctly is the winner.

ACTIVITIES FOR TEACHING DIRECTIONAL CONCEPTS

Right and left side of body

Understanding the concept of right and left will be a helpful tool for the child when practicing both asanas and pranayama. Knowing their right and left also increases body awareness and can support coordinating movements in the body. It can be common for children with motor coordination difficulties to favor one side of the body over the other, developing more strength on one side and weakness on the other side. Yoga supports balance of the physical body by incorporating poses using both the left and right sides of the body. When the body is balanced, muscles and muscle activities tend to be more balanced, in turn supporting motor activity and coordination. Subsequently, using both sides of the body supports whole brain communication by accessing both the left and right sides of the brain.

USING COLORS

Many children with special needs learn visually and are more apt to retain information when concepts are taught by connecting them to colors or images. Teaching the concept of left and right through the use of color provides a visual reference for the child when accessing left and right sides of their body.

Teaching right and left with the use of color:

Red—Right

Lavender—Left

Use red and lavender-colored stickers for right hand and left hand or use colored rubber wristbands for right and left hand. If a child exhibits tactile defensiveness towards having stickers or wrist/ankle bracelets on their skin, place the colored stickers on the right and left sleeve of their clothing.

MAKE YOUR OWN WRISTBANDS OR ANKLE BANDS
Concepts learned

▷ left and right

▷ colors

▷ counting

▷ fine motor skills

You will need

▷ red pipe cleaners

▷ lavender pipe cleaners

▷ red plastic beads

▷ lavender plastic beads

Instructions for activity

1. Have child get one red pipe cleaner and one lavender pipe cleaner.
2. Have child count out 10 red plastic beads and 10 lavender plastic beads.
3. Have child string red beads on red pipe cleaner.
4. Have child string lavender beads on lavender pipe cleaner.

If desired make two lavender bands and two red bands so the child can wear a wristband and ankle band on each side.

Top and bottom, up and down

Simply practicing yoga poses and incorporating the concept of top, bottom, up and down will support the child in increasing their understanding of directional concepts. Movement and kinesthetic activities along with language will support learning and memory of concepts. As you practice the poses with the child encourage him/her to tap the *top* of their head or the *bottom* of their feet. Have the child do the elevator breath described in Chapter 4 (see page 55) to practice the concept of up and down, starting their hands at their feet, moving their hands *up* above the head, while breathing their breath in, then moving hands back *down* to feet while breathing their breath out. Several poses suggested in Chapter 6 incorporate the concept of up and down, such as river, frog and cobra. Pre-teaching body parts and directional concepts and integrating the concepts throughout the child's practice will help the child develop a greater sense of body awareness, a connection to their own body parts and a greater understanding of how and where their bodies move.

4

PRANAYAMA (BREATHING AND BREATH AWARENESS) AND GUIDED IMAGERY

Pranayama or breathing is perhaps one of the most important components to teaching yoga to children with special needs. In order to make the connection between breathing and how it affects our physiological and emotional states, it's necessary to understand how the autonomic nervous system works. The autonomic nervous system is divided into two branches, the sympathetic and parasympathetic nervous systems.

SYMPATHETIC NERVOUS SYSTEM

The sympathetic nervous system regulates the more physical response such as responding to emergency or "perceived" emergency situations or physical exercise. When we experience anxiety, worry or fear our body perceives this as there being a threat, then activating the sympathetic nervous system. When the sympathetic nervous system is activated, the heart rate increases and less blood moves towards the digestive and excretory organs because the blood is being pumped more rapidly to the muscles of the limbs, preparing the body for fight or flight. As the heart rate increases, our breathing is also affected. When we are in the fight or flight mode, our breathing becomes accentuated and we typically move into chest breathing to prepare for more physical activity. If our bodies do not actually exert themselves through physical activity, hyperventilation or very rapid breathing may occur. This rapid breathing or hyperventilation exacerbates our emotional and physical response and can then result in a panic attack also known as an anxiety attack. Because many children with special needs may experience greater amounts of anxiety worry or fear, a heightened sensitivity to their environment and difficulty expressing their emotions, they may reside perpetually in the sympathetic nervous system (the fight/flight response). When the body becomes over-stressed and the sympathetic nervous system is in over-drive, in a constant state of fight or flight, there can be negative effects on our bodies, our moods and our behaviors.

Negative effects of being over-stressed

Physical:

- muscle tension or pain
- headaches
- fatigue
- insomnia
- digestive problems
- autoimmune conditions
- weakened immune systems
- heart problems
- back and neck pain
- ulcers
- diabetes

Emotional:

- anxiety
- restlessness
- lack of motivation
- difficulty focusing
- irritability or anger
- sadness or depression

Behavioral:

- over-eating or under-eating
- angry outbursts

- social withdrawal

- conflict with others

- obsessive-compulsive behaviors

PARASYMPATHETIC NERVOUS SYSTEM

The parasympathetic nervous system (rest and renew response) is involved in controlling resting activities such as slowing the heart rate, aiding in digestion and activating the cleansing process in the body (Rama, Balentine and Hymes 2011). Focused breathing or mindful breathing aids in moving into more of a diaphragmic breathing. Diaphragmic breathing slows the heart rate, which in turn evens out the blood flow in the body, promoting improved circulation and better digestion. Slowed, deeper, more rhythmic breathing allows us to tap into the parasympathetic nervous system, improving the overall functioning in our body. Pranayama is a necessary and key component to the practice of yoga. As described earlier, pranayama stimulates the parasympathetic nervous system, which is responsible for activating the relaxation response in our bodies. Children with special needs who experience high levels of anxiety over-stimulate their sympathetic nervous systems and under-stimulate their parasympathetic nervous systems, which can have a drastic impact on their overall health and wellbeing. Children with over-amped sympathetic nervous systems develop habitual stress responses in their bodies. This habitual stress response contributes to illnesses and health problems such as autoimmune disorders, digestive problems, insomnia, joint pain, muscle aches and a variety of other health issues. This habitual stress response also exacerbates anxiety and can contribute to obsessive-compulsive behaviors. The practice of pranayama offers a variety of emotional and physical benefits, including:

- strengthens respiratory and immune systems

- reduces stress

- energizes and increases alertness to the body and brain

- calms the nervous system (activates the parasympathetic nervous system)

- promotes healing on emotional, physical and psychological levels

- supports brain/body connection

- increases oxygen flow to brain and body

- supports healthy digestion

▶   encourages mindfulness and being connected to the present

▶   supports healthy sleep patterns.

Mindful breathing draws attention to the breath, which helps to draw attention away from the thoughts or emotions that are anxiety provoking. Many children with special needs may become fixated on an idea, a worry, a fear or other thoughts that cause anxiety. These repetitive thoughts and worries can lead to acting out with obsessive-compulsive behaviors. The practice of pranayama or mindful breathing brings the child's attention to their breath, allowing them to focus on something other than the triggering event or thought that may have initially brought about feelings of anxiety. When a child learns to control his or her breathing, the amount of oxygen in the body increases, encouraging the body to function at its optimal level. When oxygen levels increase, muscles and organs such as the brain function more efficiently. Children with special needs can often exhibit extremely high arousal states or very low arousal states. They may present themselves as being over-active, having difficulty being still or calm or underactive, being sluggish or sleepy. Various forms of breathing can either relax or stimulate the brain and body. Mindful breathing can support the child in connecting more to their body, increasing mind–body connection and awareness. Children with special needs can be taught to self-monitor and self-regulate their arousal states by learning to connect specific breaths to specific arousal states. The immense physical and emotional benefits that come with learning to breathe mindfully will last throughout the child's life and will support the child in developing a greater sense of wellbeing, promoting a happier, calmer and healthier lifestyle.

Visualization and guided imagery are both forms of meditation, with the intent to bring the mind and body to a state of deep relaxation. We learn best when our minds are in a more relaxed state. Scientists have done specific research on the effects of meditation and deep relaxation on brain waves (Bilioteca Pleyades). Just as we can see wave patterns on a heart monitor, scientists are able to monitor patterns of the brain through and EEG (electro-encephalograph). Typically the left and right brain waves are independent, peaking separately. Studies have shown that during meditation or deep relaxation, the left and right brain work together in synchronicity, peaking at the same time. Scientists now believe that this "synchronizing" of brain wave patterns lends to more clarity of mind and optimal functioning of the brain.

Visualization and meditation techniques are often taught simultaneously with breathing techniques. The idea is that we can visualize letting go of something (with the exhale) or breathing something in to our energy space (with the inhale).

Visualization strategies can also be used as a fun way to get a child motivated and excited about practicing various forms of breathing. Many of the breathing and visualization strategies outlined in this book are geared towards helping the child with regulation of emotions, calming the body, energizing the brain, releasing negative energy or emotions, focus and concentration. Guided imagery is a helpful approach to encouraging imagination and visualization while practicing yoga poses and breath. The adult can use and encourage descriptive language to help the child visualize a scene, a specific animal, color, feeling or emotion to support the child in tapping into the part of the brain that is responsible for imagination and visualization. Visualization strategies can also help the child tap into their five senses (sight, sound, touch, taste and smell) to support memory and learning. In *Spinning Inward: Using Guided Imagery with Children for Learning, Creativity & Relaxation* (1987), Murdoch discusses the role our senses play in memory and learning. She concludes that children can more easily access information and memories when they are connected to a sensory experience. She describes how using imagery and visualization increases memory, creativity and relaxation. Many children with disabilities identified in this book may struggle with imagination and visualizing spoken words. The incorporation of visuals and teaching strategies outlined earlier in the book will assist the child in having an image to draw upon while practicing the breathing techniques. This will also support them in retaining the information for future practice.

TEACHING BREATHING

Note: It is suggested that the inhale breaths for the breathing strategies in this chapter and the following chapters are through the nose rather than the mouth. Encourage the child to keep their lips sealed while breathing in.

Mouth breathing—Inhaling through the mouth can elevate blood pressure, increase respiratory problems, develop patterns of chest breathing rather than diaphragmic breathing; deplete carbon dioxide levels, reduce blood circulation; worsen asthma and sleep apnea and deprive brain, heart and other organs in the body of optimal oxygenation.

Nose breathing—filters, humidifies and moisturizes the air coming into the lungs. Inhaling through the nose can support slower, more diaphragmic breathing; support healthy and cleaner respiration; increase oxygenation to heart, brain and other organs.

BALLOON BELLY (ABDOMINAL BREATHING)

Pre-pose preparation

Use a balloon to show an example of balloon belly. Blow the balloon up and tell the child they are going to turn their belly into a balloon. Hold the balloon in front of your belly to show a visual of belly puffing up. Use a picture of a balloon to show the child in future sessions as a visual tool. Ask the child to picture their balloon. See the color of your balloon. Watch the balloon fill up as you inhale. Watch the balloon empty as you exhale. Listen to the sound of the air filling up your balloon and emptying with your breath.

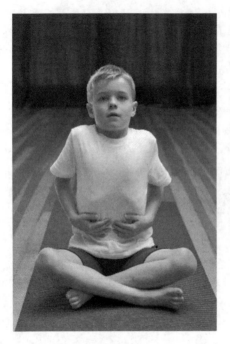 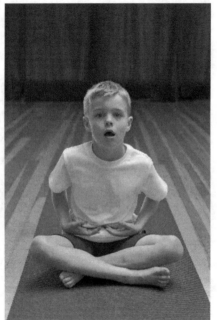

Instructions for child

1. Sit cross-legged or for more relaxation child can lie down.
2. Put both hands on belly.
3. Close lips.
4. Breathe air into balloon belly (through nose), make belly puff up like a balloon.
5. Breathe out (exhale)—let air out of balloon.
6. Repeat 4–5 times.

Benefits

Awareness of breath, relaxation, visualization, digestion.

BEE BREATH

Pre-pose preparation

Show the child a picture of a bee. Ask the child what color the bee is. Have the child close their eyes and picture the bee in their mind. Feel the soft fuzzy bee. See the bee buzzing around a beautiful flower. Listen to the sound of the bee in your breath.

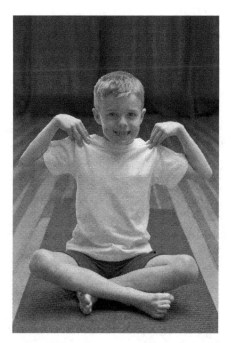

Instructions for child

1. Sit straight up in chair with hands in lap or sit cross-legged with hands in lap. (You may also suggest the child makes bee wings—fingers touching shoulders/elbows bent.)

2. Take a deep breath in (inhale deep).

3. Breathe out making a buzzing sound like a bee (bzzzz, bzzzz, bzzzz, bzzzz) until breath is empty. (If the child feels comfortable, you may suggest that they cover their ears with their palms, close their eyes and listen to the buzzing.)

4. Repeat 4–5 times.

5. Ask the child how the breath made them feel.

Benefits

Energizes the brain; eases stress and tension; helps reduce insomnia; alleviates frustration, anger and anxiety, good breath to do when child is low energy, sleepy, depressed or anxious.

UJJAYI (WAVE BREATH)

Pre-pose preparation

Talk to the child about the sound a wave makes (play an audio sound of waves in the ocean or show the child a picture of an ocean and demonstrate the sound of an ocean). Picture a blue ocean. Feel the warm water on your toes. Feel the warm sun shining on your body. Listen to the sound of the waves in your breath.

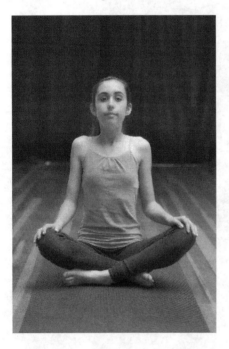
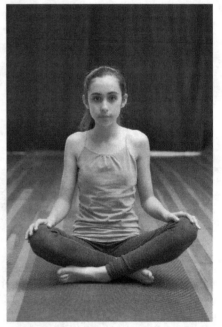

Instructions for child

1. Sit up straight in chair with hands in lap or sit cross-legged with hands in lap (you can also have the child lie down on their mat).

2. Zip lips closed (model zipping lips closed).

3. Breathe in through nose.

4. Keep lips closed.

5. Breathe out through nose.

6. Repeat 4–5 times.

Benefits

Soothes nervous system; relaxes mind and body; improves sleep.

BUNNY BREATH

Pre-pose preparation

Show picture of a bunny sniffing vegetables. Tell child to imagine being a bunny in a garden. See the colors of the vegetables and fruit in the garden. Smell the scent of the vegetables and fruit. Taste a vegetable or fruit. Is it crunchy or sweet?

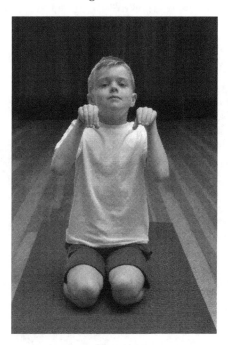
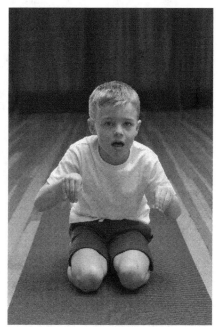

Instructions for child

1. Sit on heels or edge of chair.

2. Make bunny paws with hands.

3. Sniff the vegetables in the garden (child sniffs quickly with nose sniff, sniff, sniff, sniff, sniff until lungs are full).

4. Breathe out—haaaaaa (like a sound you would make after smelling something good).

5. Repeat 4–5 times.

Benefits
Calms the mind; energizes the brain; cleanses; alleviates frustration, anger and anxiety.

THREE-PART BREATH
Pre-pose preparation
Pre-teach three body parts where child will be breathing air into (belly, ribs, upper chest). Have child place hands on belly, then front of ribs and then upper chest just below collarbones. Recite and repeat 4–5 times, "belly," "ribs" and "chest" as the child places hands on the region. Feel the belly fill with air. Feel the ribs fill with air. Feel the chest fill with air.

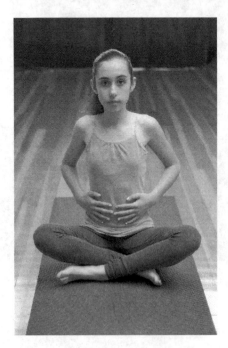 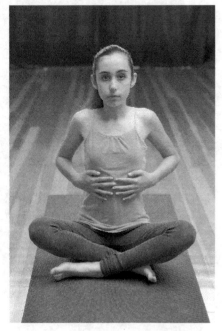

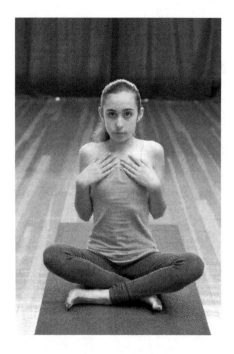

Instructions for child

1. Sit cross-legged or on the edge of a chair (you may also have the child lie down on their back).

2. Sit up tall.

3. Close lips.

4. Hands on belly.

5. Inhale—breathe air into belly through nose (make belly puff out).

6. Exhale—breathe out through nose.

7. Hands on ribs.

8. Inhale—breathe air into ribs through nose (make ribs puff out).

9. Exhale—breathe out through nose.

10. Hands on chest.

11. Inhale—breathe air into chest through nose (make chest puff out).

12. Exhale—breathe out through nose.

13. Repeat 2–3 times.

Benefits

Bring awareness to front side of body; relaxes mind and body; oxygenates bloodstream; cleanses lungs; supports digestion.

OPEN MOUTH BREATH

Pre-pose preparation

Teach where lungs are. Show a picture of lungs and talk about how they are like balloons. Put hands on chest and demonstrate full breath in—filling up lungs, chest expanding and hands pushing out. Breathe breath out and show how hands come in towards body.

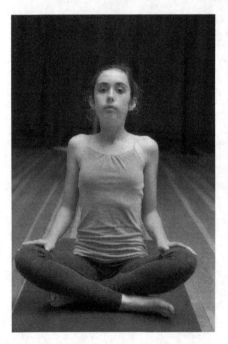 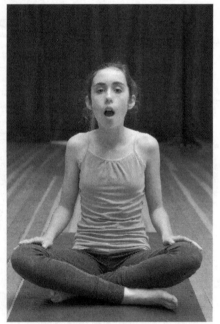

Instructions for child

1. Sit cross-legged or on edge of chair.
2. Sit up tall.
3. Breath in deep through nose, fill up lungs.
4. Breathe out through mouth (make haaaaaaa sound).
5. Repeat 4–5 times.

Benefits

Increases relaxation; releases nervous tension; increases lung capacity.

ELEVATOR BREATH

Pre-pose preparation

Show a picture of an elevator or a video of an elevator moving up and down. Tell the child "Let's make our bodies and breath move up and down like an elevator. I am going to count the floors as your elevator comes up and goes down."

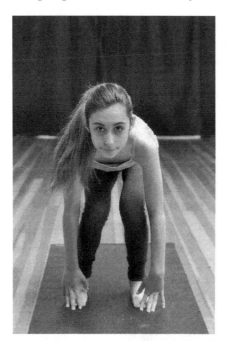
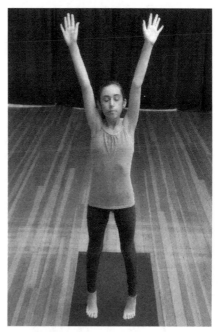

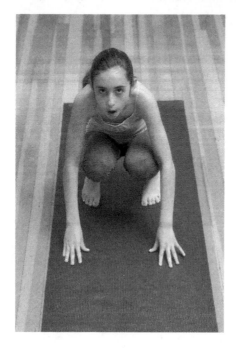

Instructions for child

1. Crouch down, fingers on mat.
2. Inhale through nose, slowly coming up to count of 1–2–3.
3. Come onto tippy toes (can modify and stay flat on feet).
4. Stretch arms up to sky.
5. Exhale through mouth, bring elevator down 3–2–1.
6. Repeat 3–4 times (option to increase the count each time telling the child, "we are going to go up one more floor on the elevator" to increase elongation of breath, ending with a count of 5).

Benefits

Increases relaxation; relieves nervous tension; increases lung capacity.

ALTERNATE NOSTRIL BREATHING

Pre-pose preparation

Note: the finger placement is modified from the traditional Alternate nostril breathing in order to simplify the finger coordination. Teach child thumb and pointer finger prior to doing the breath. If necessary place a sticker on thumb and use a piece of pipe cleaner to wrap around the pointer fingers like a ring to identify which fingers the child should use for the breath. Red sticker and pipe cleaner for Right, lavender sticker and pipe cleaner for Left. Teach child what a nostril is. "The nostrils are the two holes in our nose." Point to nostrils in nose. "We have a left nostril and a right nostril."

Instructions for child
Right hand (red for right, see page 40)

1. Press right thumb on right nostril.
2. Inhale (breathe in) through left nostril.
3. Remove right thumb.
4. Press pointer finger on left nostril.
5. Exhale (breathe out) through right nostril.

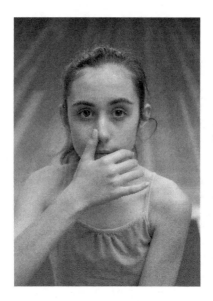 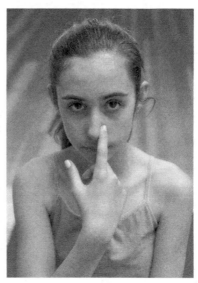

Left hand (lavender for left, see page 40)

1. Press left thumb on left nostril.
2. Inhale (breathe in) through right nostril.
3. Remove left thumb.
4. Press left pointer finger on right nostril.
5. Exhale (breathe out) through left nostril.
6. Repeat both sides 2–3 times.

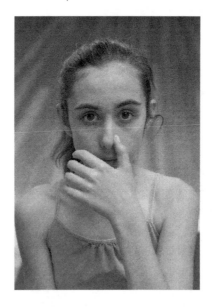 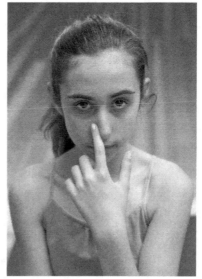

Benefits
Energizes brain; calms nervous system; improves brain function; merges the left "thinking" brain and right "feeling" brain; improves sleep; enhances relaxation.

TWO–FOUR PART BREATHING

Pre-pose preparation
Pictures or PECs with colors and emotions can be made in advance to use as visual cues for children who need more visual support.

Tell the child we are going to calm our bodies with our breath. We are going to let out a negative emotion. Ask the child what color makes them feel calm or happy. Write the color and emotion down (example: blue = happy) or have child choose color picture/PEC. Ask the child what color would anger, anxiety, frustration, worry, etc. be. Write the color and emotion down (anxiety = red) or have the child choose emotions picture/PEC. Tell the child we are going to breathe in the color blue/happiness and breathe out the color red/anxiety.

Instructions for child

1. Sit up tall in a cross-legged pose, on a chair or lying down on mat.
2. Close eyes (eyes can be open if child needs more visual support for visualization).
3. Zip lips (demonstrate zipping lips together like a zipper).
4. See the color blue. See a happy face.
5. Breathe in blue/happy feelings through nose to count of two: 1–2.
6. See the color red. See an anxious/worried face.
7. Breathe out red/anxiety through nose to count of four: 1–2–3–4.
8. Encourage child to breathe all of the air/anxiety out of their body.
9. Repeat three times.
10. Breathe in blue/happiness 1–2.
11. Breathe out red/anxiety 1–2–3–4.

Benefits
Soothes the nervous system; reduces sleep disturbance, insomnia and anxiety.

PROGRESSIVE RELAXATION

This is an excellent technique to use prior to bedtime to assist with relaxation and promote better sleep. Progressive relaxation can be done on a mat, on a blanket on the floor, on a couch or in the child's bed.

Progressive relaxation is a technique used to release tension in the body. By tensing or clenching muscles in the body, one at a time, then relaxing the muscles, the body is able to release tension and move into a more relaxed and calm state. Progressive relaxation increases body awareness, supports the child in learning and connecting to body parts and helps release tension, stress and anxiety.

Pre-pose preparation

Have the child watch the adult while seated. Describe what the words clench, tense, squeeze or tighten mean. Show the child how to clench, tense, squeeze or tighten the muscles in their body (e.g., adult squeezes fingers into a fist and says, "I clench my fingers"). Count to five as you clench your fists then release fingers and say, "I relax my fingers." Repeat one or two more examples with different body parts for the child. Soothing music turned down low may be helpful in creating a calm and relaxing environment.

Instructions for child

1. Lie on back.
2. Feet wide apart.
3. Arms wide apart.
4. Close eyes and squeeze them tight for "1–2–3–4–5."
5. Relax eyes.
6. Smile with lips closed for "1–2–3–4–5."
7. Relax lips.
8. Squeeze fingers tight in a fist for "1–2–3–4–5."
9. Relax fingers.
10. Squeeze elbows in tight to side of body for "1–2–3–4–5."
11. Relax arms.
12. Shrug shoulders to ears and hold for "1–2–3–4-5."
13. Relax shoulders.

14. Tighten belly muscles for "1–2–3–4–5."

15. Relax belly muscles.

16. Squeeze butt muscles tight for "1–2–3–4–5."

17. Relax butt muscles.

18. Squeeze legs together for "1–2–3–4–5."

19. Relax legs.

20. Clench toes and hold "1–2–3–4–5."

21. Relax toes.

22. Allow child to rest in savasana for 1–5 minutes (or longer if the child desires).

Benefits

Relieves muscular tension and muscle spasms; decreases anxiety; relieves insomnia and fatigue; soothes the nervous system; supports healthy digestion. Visualization or guided imagery can be used to promote prolonged relaxation after tensing and relaxing muscles in the body.

Example of guided imagery

"Imagine lying on a towel at the beach. The warm sun is shining on your body. Your body is relaxed. Your towel is soft and cozy. Your body is relaxed. You hear the sound of the waves. Your body is relaxed. You feel the warmth from the sun. Your body is relaxed. You see the color of the blue waves. Your body is relaxed."

5

EMOTIONS AND COMMUNICATION

Effective language skills are essential for communicating wants and needs, expressing feelings and emotions and engaging and interacting with others around us. Language development is critical to cognitive development, learning, social interaction and emotional regulation. Language processing refers to the way human beings use words to express their feelings, thoughts and ideas and how these communications are processed and understood. Many children with special needs, particularly children with ASD, have significant difficulties with language processing as well as difficulty understanding and expressing emotions. Language processing deficits can be described as having difficulty understanding or processing language when spoken to (receptive language) and/or difficulty effectively expressing thoughts or ideas (expressive language). Some children with special needs may be identified as having *auditory processing disorder*. This disorder is characterized by having difficulty understanding and processing what is heard. This does not necessarily mean that the child has hearing loss; rather their brain does not process or interpret auditory information properly. It is thought that these difficulties arise from dysfunction in the central nervous system.

Language processing deficits can occur with speech and language difficulties, learning disabilities, attention deficits or developmental disabilities. Many children with special needs may also present with social (pragmatic) communication difficulties. Children with ASD typically have challenges in this area. Social (pragmatic) communication deficits can be characterized as having difficulty with social use of language, both verbal and non-verbal, in naturalistic contexts which affects comprehension, communication with others and social relationships. Children with language and communication deficits often struggle with word retrieval and retaining learned vocabulary in their memories. They may also struggle with putting words together to form complete sentences, decoding words and comprehending written and spoken language. Children who struggle with language and communication, particularly children with autism, may also have difficulty understanding and expressing emotions.

The ability to understand and express emotions starts from birth. Typically by the age of 12 months a child can recognize the emotion their parent is feeling by looking at the expression on their face. They begin to develop the ability to imitate language, expressions, gestures and physical movements by observing others in their environment. This ability to imitate others is an important factor in developing social skills and establishing social relationships with others. Children with autism in particular struggle with the ability to imitate others. Throughout childhood and adolescence, children with typical development continue to build empathy and self-regulation skills, recognizing the emotions and perspectives of others and how they should respond to others' subtle verbal or gestural emotional cues as well as how they should regulate and respond to their own emotions. Many children with special needs as described in this book do not follow the typical development and struggle with emotional regulation, taking the perspective of others, language and communication. Often a child with special needs may not present with language processing deficits but may struggle with limited attention span, poor self-regulation, impulsivity and difficulty with perspective taking which can directly affect their ability to communicate, express emotions effectively and develop appropriate social skills. This difficulty with expressive and receptive language, difficulty communicating emotions, impulsivity and difficulty with self-regulation often leads to challenging behavior problems such as tantrum behaviors or aggressive behaviors towards others or themselves. Imagine feeling angry, anxious or worried about something and not having the ability to effectively express or communicate those emotions. Many of the breathing strategies and activities suggested in this chapter support release and expression of emotions, development of self-monitoring and self-regulation strategies, development of language, vocabulary, social skills and communication.

RELEASE AND EXPRESSION/COMMUNICATION OF EMOTIONS, SELF-MONITORING AND SELF-REGULATION OF EMOTIONAL AND PHYSICAL STATES

Many children with special needs lack effective strategies for expressing their emotions or arousal states. They can have difficulty identifying the emotions they are feeling and connecting those feelings to changes in their physical state. They may escalate quickly when they feel frustrated, anxious, angry or upset. They often tend to "act out" their emotions in a physical manner such as breaking things, aggressing towards others, self-injurious behavior, running away, exhibiting tantrums behaviors and/or "shutting down" or isolating themselves from others. These behaviors can be an attempt to release tension in their bodies as well as to release or avoid emotions that feel difficult or uncomfortable. The breathing strategies recommended in this chapter teach the child to identify the emotion they may be feeling (communication), how it feels in their body (self-monitoring) and what breathing strategies they can use to release that emotion (self-regulation). The breathing strategies suggested in this chapter support children with special needs in using healthy outlets and strategies to communicate their emotions and release negative or uncomfortable feelings in their body.

DEVELOPMENT OF LANGUAGE, VOCABULARY, COMMUNICATION AND SOCIAL SKILLS

The use of visual cues, verbalization, visualization strategies and guided imagery supports children with special needs in developing language and vocabulary, which in turn supports communication and understanding. Connecting the poses to animals or objects and providing rich, colorful and descriptive language for guided imagery, visualization, breathing strategies and poses increases vocabulary development and encourages more language and communication. Literature supports that the more children with language or communication difficulties are exposed to pictures in their environment, the more likely they are to develop language and communication in some form, whether it be verbal or non-verbal. Pictures and visual cues enhance language memory, information processing and communication. Temple Grandin, author of *Thinking in Pictures and Other Reports from My Life with Autism*, described the importance of visual supports for processing information. Grandin stated "spatial words such as over and under had no meaning for me until I had a visual image to fix them in my memory" (1995, p.30). Repetition of language and exposure to both the words with images or imagery increases understanding and comprehension. Nanci Bell, author of *Visualizing and Verbalizing*, contributes a child's difficulty with comprehension of oral and written language to a weakness in concept imagery. Bell describes mental imagery as the primary sensory-cognitive factor necessary in order to create an imaged gestalt or "whole" picture (2007, p.10). Weakness in concept imagery can result in difficulty with reading comprehension, writing skills, critical thinking, verbal expression, oral language comprehension, conversational skills and following directions. She explains how teaching children to visualize language and verbalize what they have imagined can support them with comprehension and communication. Many children with special needs exhibit weakness with concept imagery. The poses and breath incorporated in this book include language and visualizations that encourage the use of all five senses. Children will learn vocabulary and how to picture and describe animals, colors, sounds, smells, landscapes, weather or temperature, emotions, body parts and textures. Studies have also shown that children with special needs may learn language more easily through kinesthetic and motor experiences. Harvard Professor Howard Gardner presents that we each have eight different intelligences. He designated the bodily/kinesthetic as a type of intelligence and asserts that individuals can learn with bodies or body parts through movement. He asserts that movement enhances spatial intelligence and can help develop the musical, linguistic, logical/mathematical, interpersonal and intrapersonal intelligences (Gardner 1991). Children learn experientially—through play, experimentation, exploration and discovery. The brain can actually change as a result of experience. These movement experiences support the child in learning new vocabulary, strengthening brain connections and developing communication. The movement and kinesthetic experience of yoga can support the child with whole learning, making connections to vocabulary, language and the world around them through movement of their bodies.

SETTING UP THE ENVIRONMENT

Breathing strategies can be taught in a variety of environments; however, creating a consistent space for the child to do breathing activities and express emotions will support the child in developing a routine and will allow the child to have a safe, predictable space to express themselves while exploring various breathing strategies.

Suggestions for setting up a space include:

▶ Place a chair or mat in a designated space where the child can be encouraged to go when wanting to express emotions and do breathing activities.

▶ Place laminated pictures of emotions on wall or in a designated space that child can choose to support communicating how they are feeling (angry, frustrated, worried, afraid, sad, anxious, etc.).

▶ Place laminated picture choices of animals, objects and breathing activities on the wall or designated space that correlate with emotions.

▶ If necessary, use a timer to assist the child in knowing how long they have to explore breathing activities before moving on to a new activity.

Note: The breathing strategies provided in the previous chapter can also be included in the space as options for calming or energizing breathing activities. Suggestions for pre-pose and post-pose visualization and communication are provided as an option for the adult to facilitate language, communication and imagination. Depending on communication skills, each child will vary in their ability to verbalize or provide feedback. Simply using visuals and encouraging children to explore the breathing strategies will support them in releasing tension in their body as well as uncomfortable or difficult emotions they may be feeling.

DRAGON'S BREATH
Pre-pose preparation

Show child a picture of a dragon breathing fire. Talk about how the dragon has heat in its body and needs to breathe it out. Ask the child if their body feels hot when they feel angry or frustrated. Ask the child to picture a dragon in their mind. Tell the child they are going to be a dragon and release anger or frustration from their body.

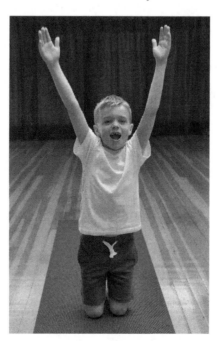 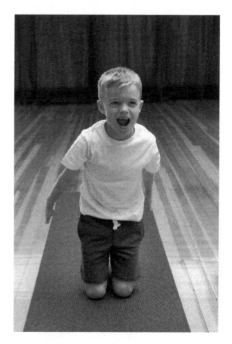

Instructions for child

1. Stand on knees on mat. Imagine heat/fire in body. Can modify by sitting cross-legged on mat or up tall in a chair.

2. Breathe in through nose and reach hands up towards ceiling (dragon wings).

3. Fly arms (dragon wings) back towards back of room.

4. Breathe fire out of mouth—sound of breath (haaaaaa!).

5. Repeat 4–5 times.

Post-pose

Ask the child to describe what their dragon looked like (what color was the dragon, what color were the wings, what did the dragon's skin feel like, etc.) and what it felt like to release the heat from their body.

Benefits

Let out anger; release tension and frustration.

VOLCANO BREATH

Pre-pose preparation

Show child a picture of a volcano erupting. Talk about how the volcano is filled with heat and is about to explode. Ask the child if they ever feel like they could explode like a volcano. Ask the child to picture a volcano erupting in their mind. Tell the child they are going to be a volcano and release anger or tension from their body.

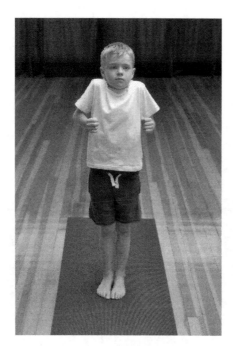 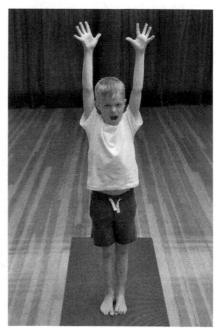

Instructions for child

1. Stand on mat. Imagine heat/fire in body.

2. Make fists at sides of body.

3. Breathe in deep through nose.

4. Reach arms up to ceiling.

5. Breathe heat out of mouth—sound of breath (haaaaaaa!).

6. Repeat 4–5 times.

Post-pose

Ask the child to describe what their volcano looked like and what it felt like to release heat and anger/tension from their body.

Benefits

Let out anger; release tension.

LION'S BREATH

Pre-pose preparation

Show the child a picture of a lion. Talk about how a lion is strong and fearless. When a lion roars it lets out its fear or worry. Ask the child what makes them feel worried or afraid. Tell the child they are going to make themselves into a lion and let out fear, worry, anxiety or anger.

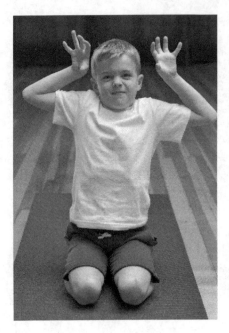 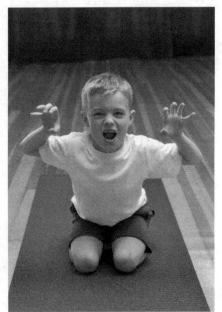

Instructions for child

1. Sit on knees with hips on heels.
2. Be a lion hiding in the bushes.
3. Bend elbows and bring hands (lion paws) up towards face.
4. Breathe in through nose.
5. Get ready to pounce.
6. Reach hands (paws) forward and roar like a lion.
7. Make lion sound (raaaaaaar!).
8. Repeat 4–5 times.

Post-pose

Ask the child to describe their lion (what did the lion's fur feel like, what color was the lion, etc.) and what it felt like to release fear, worry, anger or anxiety.

Benefits

Let out fear, worry, anxiety or anger.

CAT BREATH

Pre-pose preparation

Show a picture of a hissing cat with its back arched. Ask the child to think of something they are afraid of or makes them feel anxious.

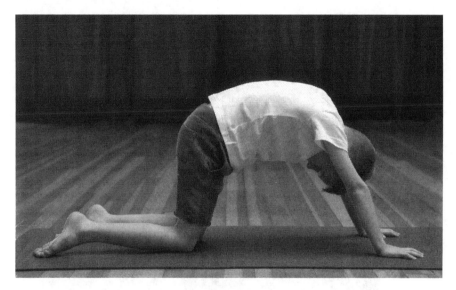

Instructions for child

1. Stand on knees.
2. Put palms on mat.
3. Back is flat like a table.
4. Breathe in deep through nose.
5. Arch back and hiss like a cat (hisssssss).
6. Breathe in through nose—straighten back.
7. Exhale—hiss like a cat.
8. Repeat 4–5 times.

Post-pose

Ask the child to describe their cat (what color was the cat, how did its fur feel, etc.) and what it felt like to let out fear or anxiety.

Benefits

Release fear or anxiety.

COBRA/SNAKE BREATH

Pre-pose preparation

Show a picture of a snake with its tongue out. Ask the child for something they are afraid of or makes them feel anxious.

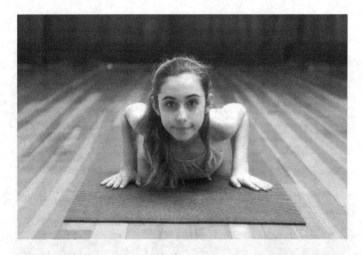

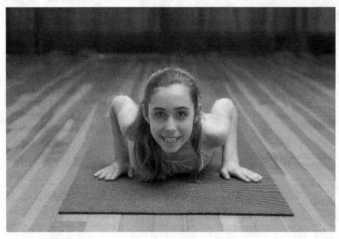

Instructions for child

1. Lie on belly.

2. Palms on mat under shoulders.

3. Breathe in through nose—lift head and shoulders off mat.

4. Breathe out—hiss like a snake (tsssssss).

5. Repeat 4–5 times.

Post-pose

Ask the child to describe their snake (what did its skin feel like, did the snake feel cold or warm, what color was the snake, etc.) and what it felt like to let out fear or anxiety.

Benefits

Release fear or anxiety.

LET IT GO BREATH

Pre-pose preparation

Have child name or draw one thing, or a list of things, that make them feel worried or anxious. The adult might suggest that the child identify an event, consistent worry or fear that they may perseverate on or focus on frequently.

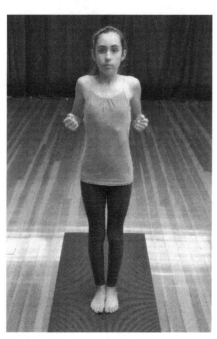 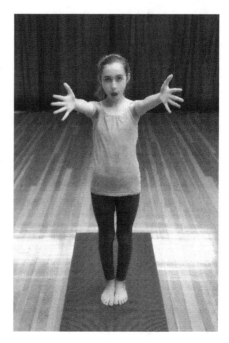

Instructions for child

1. Stand tall on mat or sit tall in chair.
2. Reach arms forward.
3. Grab worry/fear with fists.
4. Breath in through nose—pull fists to belly.
5. Breathe out, open mouth (haaaaaaa).
6. Throw worry/fear (like throwing a basketball).
7. Fingers spread wide.
8. Let it go.
9. Repeat 4–5 times.

Post-pose

Ask the child how it felt to let the worry or problem go.

Benefits

Release tension, let worry/anxiety go.

I DON'T KNOW, LET IT GO BREATH

Pre-pose preparation

Have child think of doing something that they don't know how to do or that is difficult for them. The child can draw a picture of the activity or write the word down (e.g., child draws a picture of a math problem). Talk about how it's ok if we don't know something or aren't perfect at something. When we are doing something that is difficult or we don't know how to do it, we can do this breath.

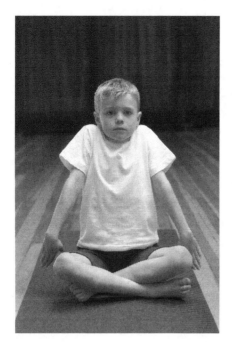 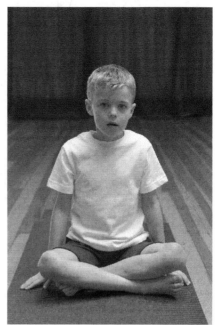

Instructions for child

1. Sit cross-legged or up tall in a chair.
2. Breathe in through nose—shrug shoulders up to ears (think of words "I don't know").
3. Breathe out—haaaaaaa (think of words "Let it go").
4. Repeat 4–5 times.

Post-pose

Ask the child how it felt to let the worry or problem go.

Benefits

Release tension, worry or fear of making mistakes.

6

ASANAS (PHYSICAL POSES)

As described in Chapter 1, "What is Yoga?", the practice of asanas (physical poses) offers many benefits to the child including strengthening the nervous system, supporting digestion, improving sleep patterns, aiding circulation and improving overall health. In addition, practicing asanas supports children with autism and special needs by improving strength and flexibility, developing body awareness, increasing balance and coordination, supporting sensory imbalances, strengthening motor skills, increasing focus and concentration, developing increased self-esteem and self-confidence and managing stress more effectively. The poses described in this chapter offer specific benefits. The benefits of each pose are provided in order to identify which poses would meet the needs of the individual child.

A NOTE ABOUT BREATHING

The child should be encouraged to breathe and continue the breath while in each pose. Specific breathing strategies are suggested for each pose. If the child is not able to perform each breath just right, simply encourage the child to breathe. Focusing on the breath will bring attention to their breathing and encourage the child not to hold their breath in the poses.

ADDITIONAL CONSIDERATIONS

Due to a child with special needs having varying degrees of difficulty with language processing, sensory input (including external sounds and noise), anxiety, possible OCD behaviors along with other acting out behaviors, it is important that the adult have knowledge and understanding of specific triggers, challenges and needs that may come up when introducing yoga to each individual child.

It is also important to know any health conditions or diagnosis the child has, as there may be specific contraindications for certain poses and breathing strategies.

RULES FOR YOGA
CHILL:

Calm voice

Have fun

In control

Listening ears

Looking eyes

What you will need:

▶ yoga mat (preferably plain—visuals on mat may be distracting or confusing)

▶ colored rubber circles

▶ pictures/visuals

▶ colored wrist-bands (see art activity—red–right, lavender–left on page 40)

Other suggested materials:

▶ yoga block

▶ calming music

▶ yoga blanket

▶ eye pillow

YOGA POSE TERMS

Seated—any poses in which the individual is sitting down.

Supine—any pose in which the individual is lying down.

Standing—any pose in which the individual is standing. Standing poses help build strength in the body and support healthy posture.

Balancing—any pose in which the individual is balancing on one foot or on one body part. Balancing poses help build strength in the body and increase focus and concentration.

Flexion—any pose in which the spine is moving into flexion (forward bending poses or lateral bending poses). Forward bending poses increase suppleness in the spine, ease tension in back and neck muscles and decrease anxiety by activating the parasympathetic nervous system to create a sense of calm and relaxation. Lateral bending postures strengthen the oblique muscles, increase flexibility in the spine and support balance.

Extension—any pose in which the spine is moving into extension (back bending poses). Back bending poses open up the front side of the body, realign the spine, support healthy posture, boost the immune system and aid in reducing depression.

Twisting—any pose in which the spine is being twisted or rotated. Twisting poses help restore the spines natural range of motion, cleanse and detoxify internal organs, support healthy digestion and improve circulation.

Inversion—any pose in which the head is below the heart. Inversion poses improve circulation by reversing the flow of blood in the body and boost the immune system. Cooling inversions suggested in this book (down dog and spider legs up the wall) reduce anxiety by activating the parasympathetic nervous system.

SETTING UP THE ENVIRONMENT

Safety

Create a safe space for the child to move around. Remove any objects from the floor that the child may step on. Allow enough space for the child to practice poses without bumping into or tripping over furniture or objects.

Boundary

Create a visual boundary for the child so they know where to stand and position their body during practice. A yoga mat is a great visual and physical boundary for the child. A rubber circle can also be a helpful tool if the pose requires the child to stand in a more specific or designated spot.

Space

Allow enough space in the environment for the child to move around and practice the poses without feeling too cramped or inhibited.

Sensory supporting

The space where the child practices should be free of bright lights, loud noises or any other factors that could be distressing to their sensory system. Soothing music can be calming and may be helpful as an auditory tool for relaxation; however, some children with sensory integration difficulties may find it distracting.

Clothing

Whenever possible have the child wear comfortable and/or loose fitted clothing. Have them wear layers of clothing that suit the temperature of the room so they are not too hot or too cold. Encourage the child to practice yoga poses barefoot. If the child does not prefer being barefoot they can wear socks, preferably non-slip ones, to practice poses.

Tools and Props

Use tools and materials suggested on page 76 whenever necessary to support the child in doing poses.

OTHER CONSIDERATIONS

Balance

If the child does a pose on one side always attempt to have them do the pose on the opposite side. Using both sides of the body supports activating the left and right hemispheres of the brain, encouraging whole brain integration and motor coordination.

Modifications and considerations

Begin by teaching seated and supine postures to children who have low muscle tone or have more severe difficulties with coordination and balance. Many children with Down syndrome may have hypermobile joints and can hyperextend their joints easily. Encourage them to bend their knees when folding forward in poses and avoid overstretching in poses. Incorporate standing postures in their yoga practice. Standing postures can help stabilize tendons and cartilage in knees and ankles. If a child is overweight or obese avoid poses where they are lying on their belly. Lying on their belly can compress their lungs and make it difficult for them to breathe easily. Always monitor a child's breath and physical response to poses. Incorporate suggestions for modifications to the pose or eliminate the pose altogether if the child is unable to breathe freely, seems to be straining too much or the pose seems too difficult for the child. Although yoga can be a complimentary support for seizure disorders, it is important to be aware if the child has a seizure disorder. Knowing how often they occur and what triggers them will help identify any poses that may be risky (e.g., balancing poses) and be prepared to respond if a seizure occurs. The use of a table, chair or wall in balancing poses can be a helpful modification to support balance and ensure safety.

Diversity

Incorporate a diversity of poses into the child's practice including seated, supine, standing, balancing, flexion, extension and inversion poses (keeping in mind modifications and considerations).

Breathing

Breathing should be encouraged with the practice of any pose. Mindful breathing brings the body into a more relaxed and focused state, which will support the child in doing the poses safely while maximizing the benefits of the pose. Specific types of breathing are suggested for each pose in the book. Although these breathing strategies are recommended, if a breath is too difficult for the child, simply focus on bringing awareness to their breath. The child should never strain while doing breathing strategies. If the breathing strategy seems too difficult or abstract, taking slow and steady open mouth inhales and exhales will still benefit the child.

Predictability

Predictability is important to many children with special needs, particularly children with autism. Not knowing what to expect or how long an activity may be can be upsetting and anxiety provoking to the child. Many children with special needs have difficulty understanding or recognizing the concept of time. Routine and predictability creates a sense of order for a child who feels less in control over their environment. Making the child's yoga practice as predictable as possible will support the child in knowing what to expect and will give them a frame of reference for what, when and how long the activity will be. Developing a predictable routine will support the child in learning the routine. Repetition and sameness supports learning, retention of information and independence.

Energizing versus calming

Be aware of poses that energize versus poses that calm. If a child has high levels of anxiety, a focus on poses that calm the nervous system would be more appropriate. Most forward bending poses help with anxiety and activating the parasympathetic nervous system. Typically more restorative poses that aid in better sleeping patterns and decrease insomnia would be best to practice prior to bedtime. Most back bending, balancing and standing poses energize the brain and body but can also aid in decreasing stress and anxiety. Energizing poses can also be good for a child who has high energy and is highly distractible since the poses require more physical exertion, concentration and focus. It can be helpful to begin with more energizing poses and end with more restorative poses if the overall desired effect is to slow the child's system down.

Descriptions of poses in this chapter provide information on whether the pose is calming or energizing along with the specific benefits of each pose. A combination of energizing and calming poses will give the child a balanced practice. Each individual child will vary in their response to poses. It is up to the adult or guide to identify how the child responds to each pose in order to develop an individualized practice that works for the child.

Timing

Be aware of timing when the child practices specific poses. Choose poses that are soothing and calming when you want the child to relax, such as prior to bedtime. Choose poses that are energizing and invigorating when you want the child to have more energy such as prior to going to school in the morning. Avoid having the child practice poses after eating. Allow for at least 1–2 hours to digest food prior to practicing yoga poses if possible. Poses should only be held for a few breaths at a time.

Energy and mood

It is important to be aware of both the adult and child's emotional energy and mood when practicing yoga. Yoga is meant to be a positive and calming experience. The emotional energy of the adult can transfer to the child during a yoga practice. The experience would be most optimal if the adult is in an emotional place to guide the child with patience and a gentle tone. If the child is resistive to the practice it may be best to suggest doing yoga at another time.

Practicing as a family unit

Yoga is not only beneficial to a child with special needs, it can also be beneficial to the family as a whole. Practicing poses and breathing strategies as a family unit will encourage and support the child in their yoga practice and will benefit the family by reducing the stress, anxiety and tension that often comes with the challenges of living with a child with special needs. Calm, peaceful and relaxing time together as a family can be healing and bonding. Playing yoga games together as a family can be time spent having fun, interacting and enjoying each other. Parents, siblings and family members of children with special needs can benefit physically and emotionally from practicing yoga as well!

SEQUENCING OF POSES

Below is a general guide for sequencing yoga poses when developing a yoga routine for a child with special needs. This guide is simply a suggestion and can be adapted to meet the specific preferences and needs of each individual child. Children with special needs will benefit from practicing any yoga poses that are at their level of ability and may gravitate towards one pose more than another. Being in tune to the child's response to each pose will help the adult develop a sequence that is motivating and enjoyable for the child. The adult will want to take factors into consideration such as energy level, mood, time of day, ability, preference, modifications and considerations, etc., as described in the beginning of this chapter when creating a sequence for the child.

1. *Seated or supine*: It is best to begin the yoga practice seated or lying down (supine). This is a good time to bring focus to mindful breathing, using the breathing strategies suggested in Chapter 4.

2. *Spine awakening*: Spine awakening poses such as down dog and cat/cow will begin to gently stretch the spine and awaken the body.

3. *Sun salutations*: Sun salutations warm the muscles in the body and prepare them for deeper stretching poses. They are also invigorating and energizing. Flowing from one pose to the next to supports sensory processing.

4. *Standing and balancing poses*: Standing and balancing poses strengthen the muscles in the legs, help develop core stability, increase focus and concentration and support sensory processing.

5. *Standing forward folding poses*: Standing forward folding poses can be alternated with standing and balancing poses. This movement from standing to forward bending supports sensory processing and invigorates and calms the body at the same time.

6. *Gentle back bends*: Gentle back bends such as shark, cobra and bridge pose can be both rejuvenating and calming.

7. *Seated forward folding poses*: Seated forward folding poses will support the child's body in slowing down and preparing for rest.

8. *Seated or supine twisting poses*: Seated or supine twisting poses balance out the spine from flexion and extension movements and activate the digestive process to support healthy digestion.

9. *Tensing muscles prior to relaxation*: Encouraging the child to tense their muscles in the body will prepare them for relaxation (e.g., sponge pose, squeezing the body tight like a sponge to release any tension, stress or anxiety from the body and progressive relaxation).

10. *Savasana (resting pose)*: This is the final resting pose that encourages relaxation, stillness and activation of the parasympathetic nervous system or resting system.

11. *Fetal pose*: Having the child roll onto side in the fetal position supports a slow and calm transition out of their yoga practice in order to maintain activation of the parasympathetic nervous system.

12. *Seated and closing of practice*: Having the child come out slowly from a lying down position will support their nervous system in maintaining a calm state.

13. *Namaste*: Depending on preference, the adult may choose to close the practice with Namaste, as described in the beginning of the book (see page 16) or may have a different preference for ending the practice. Reminding the child of their unique light and what is special about them promotes self-love and nurturing feelings towards themselves.

PHYSICAL POSES/ASANAS

Relaxing/calming poses

Relaxing and calming poses activate the parasympathetic nervous system, bringing the body and mind to a calmer, more relaxed state. Forward folding poses such as rag doll, rabbit and turtle, as well as more restorative poses such as spider legs up the wall, fetal pose and savasana, slow the body down and prepare the body for rest. Relaxing and calming poses support digestion, slow the heart rate and allow the muscles and organs of the body to relax and repair.

CHILD'S POSE (BALASANA)

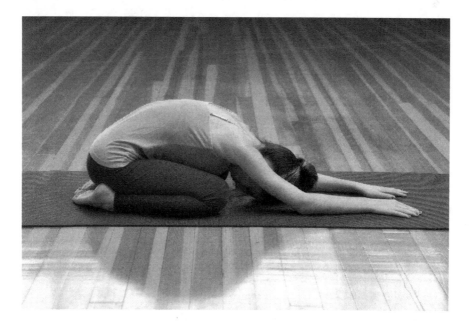

Instructions for pose

1. Kneel on mat.
2. Sit back on heels.
3. Spread knees wide apart.
4. Reach fingers up to the sky.
5. Bring forehead to mat.
6. Stretch fingers to front of mat.

7. Palms on mat.

8. Breathe.

Breath

▷ ujjayi

▷ open mouth breaths

Benefits

Releases tension in the back, shoulders and chest; improves digestion; lengthens and stretches the spine; gently stretches the hips, thighs and ankles; improves circulation; stretches muscles, tendons and ligaments in the knee; calms the mind and body; helps alleviate stress and anxiety; encourages strong and steady breathing.

Body awareness

▷ heels

▷ knees

▷ hips

▷ forehead

▷ arms

▷ palms

▷ fingers

Visualization

Think of a calm, soothing color or place.

Modifications

Block or blanket under forehead, blanket under knees, knees spread wide apart or together, blanket in creases behind knees.

ROCK

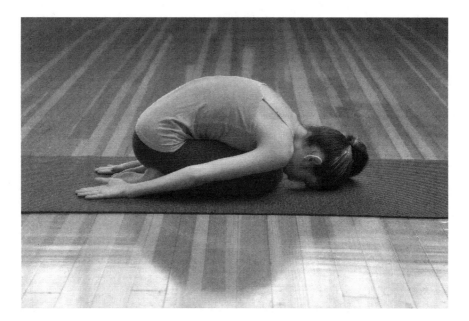

Instructions for pose

1. Stand on knees on mat.
2. Sit back on heels.
3. Knees together.
4. Bring forehead to mat.
5. Reach fingers back towards heels.
6. Relax arms to side.
7. Breathe.

Breath

▷ ujjayi

▷ open mouth breath

Benefits

Stretches the hips, thighs and ankles; relaxes the muscles on the front of the body; gently stretches the muscles of the back torso; reduces stress and fatigue; centers, calms and soothes the brain and body; normalizes circulation; strengthens immune system.

Body awareness

▷ heels

▷ knees

▷ hips

▷ forehead

▷ arms

Visualization

Imagine being a rock sitting in the grass, the warm sun shining down on you, a quiet, calm rock, warm from the sun.

Modifications

Allow hips to lift off heels if needed, place a folded blanket under knees.

CROSS-LEGGED (SUKHASANA)

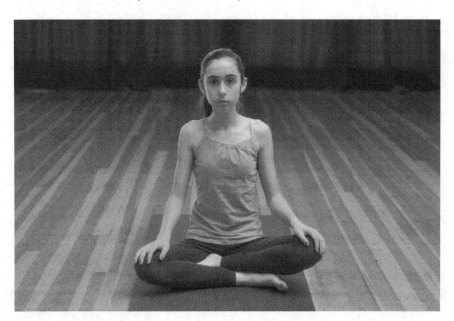

Instructions for pose

1. Sit on mat.
2. Cross legs.
3. Sit up tall.
4. Relax shoulders.
5. Palms face down on knees.
6. Breathe 5–6 breaths.

Breath

▷ falling out breath

▷ ujjayi breath

▷ balloon belly breath

Benefits

Calms the brain; helps with focus and concentration; strengthens the back; stretches the knees and ankles.

Body awareness

▷ ankles

▷ knees

▷ spine

▷ shoulders

▷ top of head

Visualization

Think of something that makes you feel calm and happy.

Modifications

Sit on a folded blanket.

RAG DOLL (UTTANASANA)

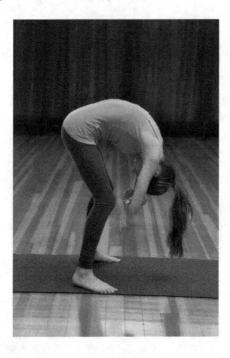

Instructions for pose

1. Stand tall on mat.
2. Inhale—reach arms to sky.
3. Exhale—bend forward.
4. Hold elbows.
5. Nod head yes.
6. Shake head no.

Breath

▷ ujjayi

▷ open mouth breath

Benefits

Calms the brain and helps relieve stress and anxiety; stimulates liver and kidneys; stretches the hamstrings, calves and hips; strengthens the thighs and knees; improves digestion; reduces fatigue.

Body awareness

▷ feet

▷ knees

▷ spine

▷ arms

▷ elbows

▷ fingers

Visualization

Imagine your body flopping over like a rag doll.

Modifications

Hands on chair, bend knees.

RABBIT (SHASHANKASANA)

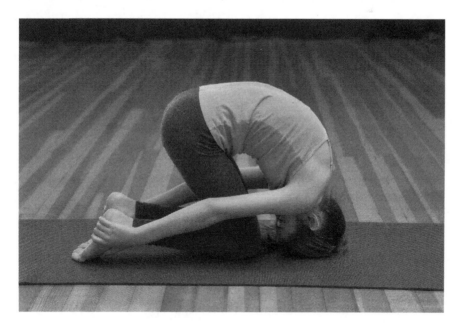

Instructions for pose

1. Stand on knees.

2. Sit back on heels.

3. Lower top of head to mat.

4. Lift hips (bunny tail) high towards sky.

5. Breathe.

Breath

▷ ujjayi

▷ open mouth

Benefits

Stretches hips, thighs, ankles, chest, shoulders and arms; relieves tension, stress and fatigue; calms the mind.

Body awareness

▷ knees

▷ heels

▷ top of head

▷ hips

Visualization

Imagine being a rabbit, curling up in a ball, lifting its tail to the sky.

Modifications

Lift hips only slightly.

TURTLE (KURMASANA)

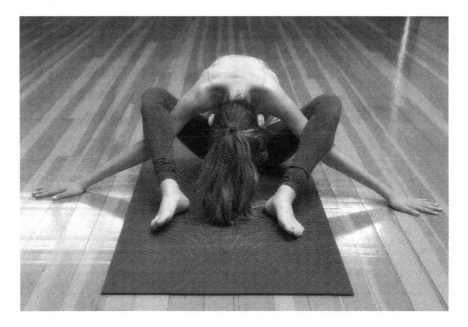

Instructions for pose

1. Sit on mat.
2. Spread legs wide.
3. Breathe in.
4. Lean forward and stretch arms forward on mat.
5. Bend knees a little.
6. Walk hands underneath knees (right under right, left under left).
7. Forehead can come onto mat.
8. Breathe.

Breath

▷ ujjayi

▷ open mouth

Benefits

Stretches hips, groin, hamstrings, shoulders and upper and lower back; supports digestion; calms the mind.

Body awareness

- ▷ feet
- ▷ knees
- ▷ palms
- ▷ arms
- ▷ back
- ▷ forehead

Visualization

Imagine being a turtle in its shell, slow and calm.

Modifications

Stop at step 4—stretching arms forward, bend knees more.

DOWN DOG (ADHO MUKHA SVANASANA)

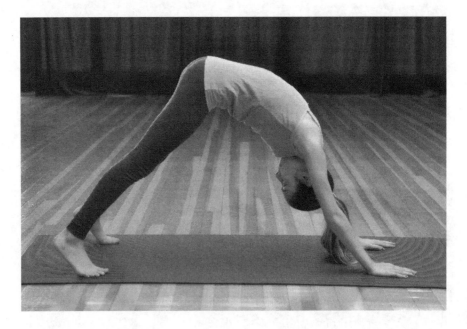

Instructions for pose

1. Sit on heels.
2. Spread fingers wide.

3. Come to hands and knees.

4. Fingers spread wide on mat.

5. Inhale.

6. Tuck toes.

7. Exhale.

8. Lift hips up to sky.

9. Look back at heels.

10. Breathe.

Breath

▷ ujjayi

▷ open mouth

Benefits

Stretches hands, wrists, shoulders, hamstrings, calves and arches of feet; strengthens arms and legs; supports digestion; calms brain, relieves stress and anxiety; improves circulation and energizes the body.

Body awareness

▷ palms

▷ arms

▷ head

▷ hips

▷ feet

▷ heels

Visualization

Imagine a dog stretching, lifting its tail high.

Modifications

Bend knees, puppy pose (if down dog is too difficult).

PUPPY (UTTANA SHISHOSANA)

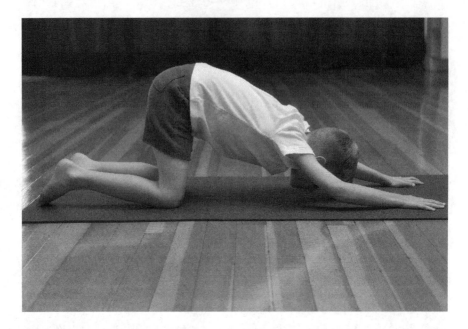

Instructions for pose

1. Come to hands and knees.
2. Inhale.
3. Exhale.
4. Bring elbows to mat.
5. Bring forehead to mat.
6. Lift hips high.
7. Breathe.

Breath

▷ ujjayi

▷ open mouth

Benefits

Stretches the spine and shoulders; calms the mind; supports digestion; helps alleviate stress and anxiety.

Body awareness

▷ forehead

▷ shoulders

▷ knees

▷ hips

Visualization

Imagine a puppy stretching its body, tail lifting to the sky.

Modifications

Puppy pose is a modification for down dog pose.

BUTTERFLY (BADDHA KONASANA)

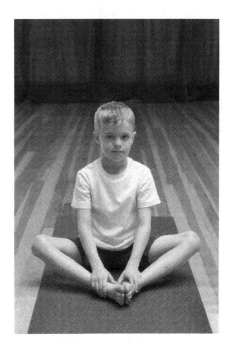 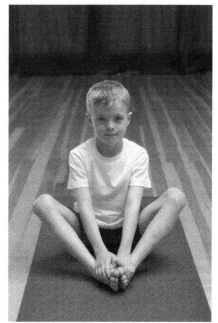

Instructions for pose

1. Sit on mat.

2. Bring bottoms of feet to touch each other.

3. Hold ankles or feet.

4. Sit up tall.

5. Inhale—lift knees up.

6. Exhale—bring knees down.

7. Flap your butterfly wings.

8. Repeat 5–6 times.

Breath

▷ ujjayi

▷ open mouth

Benefits

Stretches inner thighs, groins and knees; improves digestion and circulation; helps relieve mild depression, anxiety and fatigue; helps with asthma symptoms.

Body awareness

▷ bottoms of feet

▷ knees

▷ belly

▷ spine

▷ shoulders

▷ hands

Visualization

Imagine a butterfly flapping its wings. Think of what color your butterfly is. Imagine your butterfly flying in the sky.

Modifications

Bring bent knees higher up from ground, sit against a wall, do pose lying down on mat.

GIRAFFE (PRASARITA PADOTTANASANA)

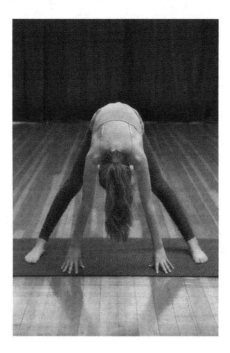

Instructions for pose

1. Stand sideways on mat.
2. Spread legs wide (feet parallel to each other).
3. Reach arms out to side.
4. Inhale deeply.
5. Exhale—lean body forward.
6. Bring hands to mat.
7. Breathe.

Breath

▷ ujjayi

▷ open mouth

Benefits

Strengthens and stretches inner thighs, hamstrings and spine; improves circulation; calms the brain; helps alleviate anxiety; combats fatigue, headaches and mild depression.

Body awareness

▷ feet

▷ legs

▷ spine

▷ head

▷ hands

Visualization

Imagine a giraffe with its long legs spread wide bending down to drink water from a pond.

Modifications

Bend knees, place a soft block or folded blanket underneath head to increase calming effect. Do pose with back against the wall.

SPONGE

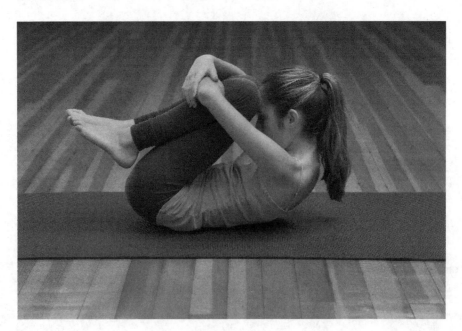

Instructions for pose

1. Lie on back.
2. Bring knees toward body.
3. Wrap arms around knees.
4. Bring forehead to knees.
5. Squeeze knees tight to body—hold for a count of four.
6. Exhale—lay body flat on mat (arms and legs spread wide).

Breath

Hold breath while tensing, open mouth to release.

Benefits

Releases tension in body; relaxes the muscles in the body; soothes the nervous system.

Body awareness

▷ arms

▷ knees

▷ forehead

Visualization

Imagine your body as a sponge. Squeeze worry, tension or anxiety out of your sponge.

SELF-HUG (BOTH SIDES)

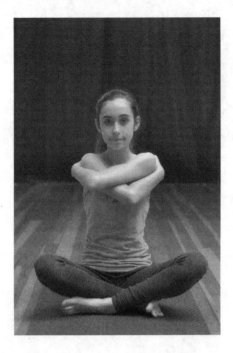

Instructions for pose

1. Sit cross-legged (or stand tall).
2. Reach fingers forward.
3. Cross right elbow over left.
4. Bring fingers to shoulder blades.
5. Inhale—squeeze and hug yourself tight.
6. Exhale—relax hug and say, "I love me."
7. Repeat inhale—squeeze and exhale—relax 2–3 times.
8. Repeat on opposite side—left elbow over right.

Breath

▷ ujjayi
▷ open mouth

Benefits

Relieves tension in shoulders, upper back and neck; calms the mind; encourages self-love.

Body awareness

- arms
- shoulders

Visualization

When you hug your arms around yourself think of love and happy feelings.

RIVER

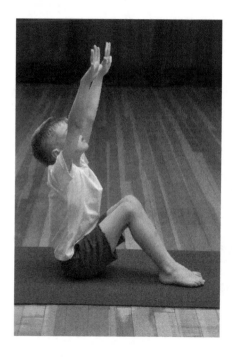 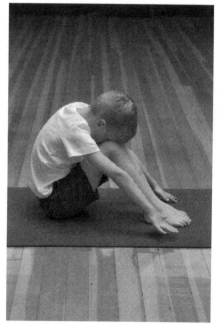

Instructions for pose

1. Sit on mat with legs straight.
2. Bend knees, bottoms of feet on mat.
3. Breathe in, reach fingers up to the ceiling.

4. Breathe out, fold forwards, arms down bring fingers down to ground, plams facing floor.

5. Forehead on knees.

6. Repeat 4–5 times.

Breath

▷ ujjayi

▷ open mouth breath

Benefits

Strengthens core; stretches back and shoulders; relieves tension and stress.

Body awareness

▷ knees

▷ legs

▷ belly

▷ arms

▷ fingers

Visualization

Imagine water in a river gently rising and falling.

Modifications

Arms on ground behind back to support weight.

SPIDER LEGS UP THE WALL (VIPARITA KARANI)

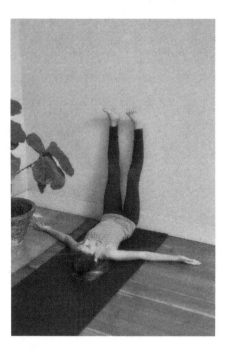

Instructions for pose

1. Sit sideways against a wall.
2. Crawl legs up wall.
3. Bring back onto mat.
4. Spread arms wide.
5. Palms face up to sky.
6. Close eyes.
7. Breathe.
8. Suggested time in pose is 5–10 minutes (modify time to meet needs of child).

Breath

▷ natural breathing

Benefits

Gently stretches back of legs, front torso and back of neck; improves circulation; supports digestion; helps relieve insomnia, anxiety and depression; alleviates headaches.

Body awareness

- ▷ hips
- ▷ legs
- ▷ back
- ▷ shoulders
- ▷ arms

Visualization

Imagine your legs are spider legs crawling up the wall. Think of a color that makes you feel calm.

Modifications

Place folded blanket or towel under lower back, bend knees slightly.

RESTING POSE (SAVASANA)

Doing progressive relaxation or sponge pose prior to savasana will support the child in relaxing the body prior to savasana. The adult can make the decision regarding the amount of time the child stays in savasana based on their individual needs. Recommended time is 5–10 minutes. If the child begins to get fidgety, it is a good sign that they are ready to come out of savasana. Calm music in the background may be helpful in supporting deep relaxation in savasana. Savasana is the ending pose to the yoga practice. Have the child come out of savasana by moving into fetal pose first, then sitting up.

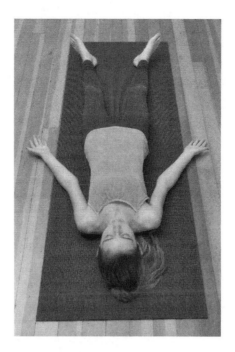

Instructions for pose

1. Lie on back.

2. Spread legs wide.

3. Spread arms wide.

4. Close eyes.

5. Relax body.

Have the child come out of savasana by moving to the fetal position first.

Breath

▷ natural breathing

Benefits

Soothes the nervous system; calms the brain; helps relieve anxiety and mild depression; reduces headache, fatigue and insomnia.

Body awareness

▷ legs

▷ arms

▷ palms

Visualization

Imagine lying in soft, warm clouds.

Modifications

Place a blanket on top of child to increase soothing and grounding effect. Place eye pillow on child's eyes to improve relaxation.

FETAL POSE (ON SIDE)

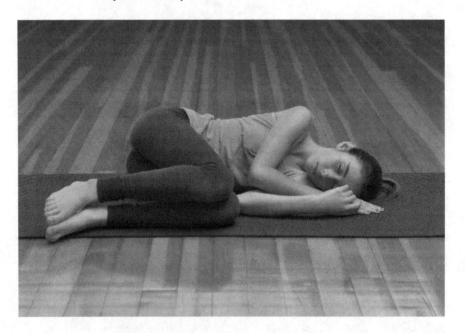

Instructions for pose

1. Lie on side (right suggested).

2. Bend knees.

3. Close eyes.

4. Breathe.

Breath

▷ natural breathing

Benefits

Calms the mind and helps alleviate anxiety; is a good transitional pose when coming out of supine poses (such as savasana) into seated pose so the child comes up slowly and maintains a state of calm.

Body awareness

▷ side

▷ shoulder

▷ knees

▷ arms

Visualization

Imagine a baby curled up, sleeping.

Modifications

Place a blanket on the child to enhance calming, relaxing effect.

Invigorating/energizing poses

Invigorating and energizing poses increase alertness, attention and focus while decreasing fatigue, stress and anxiety. Invigorating poses can calm the mind while physically energizing the brain and body at the same time. Practicing invigorating/energizing poses can provide a natural energy boost when a child is fatigued, lethargic or has low energy. These uplifting poses stimulate the circulation system and awaken the nervous system. When our bodies are stagnant for longer periods of time our energy systems can get stuck. These poses can be practiced in the morning and throughout the day to boost energy and energize the child's brain and body.

CAT/COW (MARJARYASANA/BITILASANA)

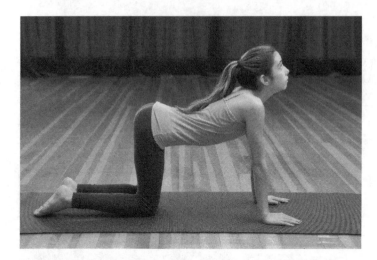

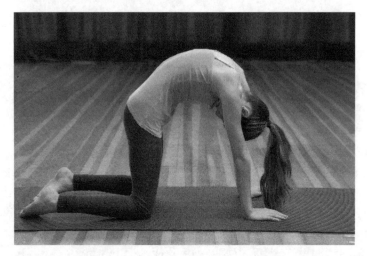

Instructions for pose

1. Stand on knees—(have child space knees hip width apart).
2. Put palms on mat (make yourself into a table). Child should have hips stacked over knees and shoulders stacked over wrists.
3. Inhale through nose—drop belly, look up.
4. Press palms into floor.
5. Arch back like a scared cat.
6. Exhale through mouth (or hiss like a scared cat).
7. Repeat 4–5 times.

Breath

Inhale through nose; exhale through mouth (or hiss like a cat).

Benefits

Stretches spine; releases tension in spine; extension and flexion of spine; opens and stretches upper back and pectoralis muscles in front; energizes the body and calms the mind.

Body awareness

- fingers spread wide
- shoulders/wrists (stacked)
- spine
- hips/knees (stacked)

Visualization

Imagine a cow in green grass, looking up at sky and a cat arching back when it hisses.

Modifications

Blanket under knees.

BOAT (NAVASANA)

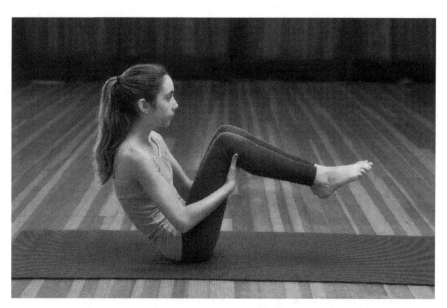

Instructions for pose

1. Sit on mat with legs straight.
2. Bend knees.
3. Hold behind knees.
4. Lift toes.
5. Lean back.
6. Sit up straight.
7. Breathe.

Breath

▷ ujjayi
▷ open mouth breath

Benefits

Strengthens hips, thighs and abdominal muscles; improves balance, coordination; improves digestion; stimulates kidneys and thyroid; develops focus and concentration.

Body awareness

▷ bottom
▷ hips
▷ belly
▷ spine
▷ back of knees
▷ feet

Visualization

Imagine a strong ship or boat sitting in the ocean.

Modifications

Palms on floor next to hips with elbows bent.

PLANK (KUMBHAKASANA)

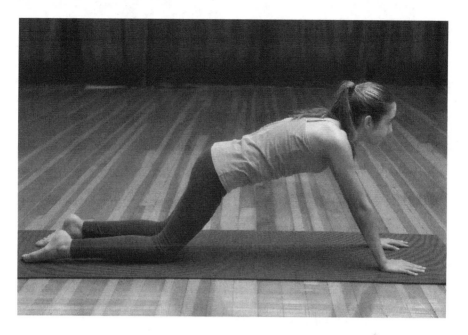

Instructions for pose

1. Lie on belly.
2. Bring palms under shoulders.
3. Spread fingers wide.
4. Inhale.
5. Lift body up with arms (like a push up).
6. Keep knees on mat.
7. Keep arms straight.
8. Pull belly button in tight.
9. Keep neck straight.
10. Breathe.

Breath

▷ ujjayi
▷ open mouth

Benefits
Strengthens upper body, chest, shoulders, arms and wrists; strengthens the core (responsible for balance).

Body awareness
▷ palms

▷ fingers

▷ arms

▷ knees

▷ belly

Visualization
Imagine a strong wooden plank on a pirates ship. Make your body into a plank.

Modifications
Folded blanket under knees. This pose is a modified version of the full plank pose.

FROG (MALASANA)

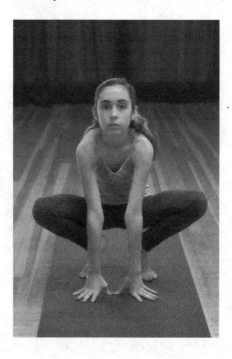

Instructions for pose

1. Squat on floor, balancing on toes.
2. Spread knees wide.
3. Hands on floor between legs.
4. Inhale—lift hips up (head comes closer to floor).
5. Exhale—come back to squat.
6. Repeat 4–5 times.

Breath

- ▷ ujjayi
- ▷ cleansing breath (inhale through nose, exhale tongue out like catching a fly on tongue)

Benefits

Strengthens and tones legs; stretches feet and ankles; stretches back torso and groins; improves heart health.

Body awareness

- ▷ toes
- ▷ heels
- ▷ knees
- ▷ hips
- ▷ spine
- ▷ hands

Visualization

Imagine a frog sitting on a lily pad getting ready to leap or jump off the lily pad.

Modifications

Sit on a block or thick book.

MOUNTAIN POSE TO MOUNTAIN PEAK (TADASANA)

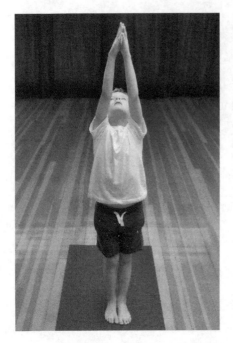 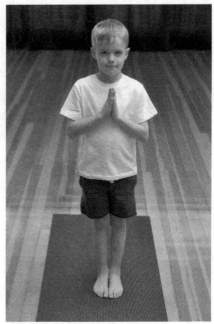

Instructions for pose

1. Stand on mat with feet together.
2. Spread toes wide.
3. Arms to side (palms facing body).
4. Inhale—stretch arms up to sky.
5. Look up.
6. Palms together at top of head.
7. Exhale—palms to chest/front of body.
8. Repeat 4–5 times.

Breath

▷ ujjayi

▷ open mouth breath

Benefits

Strengthens and tones legs, knees, ankles, lower abdomen, shoulders and neck; improves posture; increases self-esteem; supports balance and focus.

Body awareness

▷ toes

▷ feet

▷ legs

▷ belly

▷ shoulders

▷ arms

▷ palms

▷ crown of head

Visualization

Imagine standing strong and tall like a mountain.

Modifications

Feet slightly apart (hip width).

SUN SALUTATION (WAKING THE SUN) SEQUENCE: MOUNTAIN PEAK, FORWARD FOLD, PLANK, MOUNTAIN

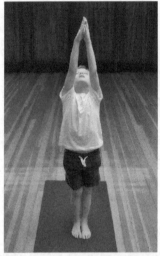
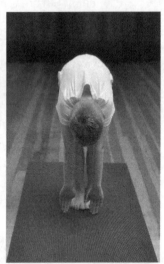
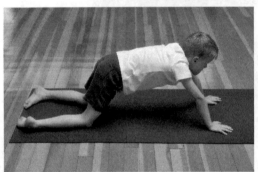
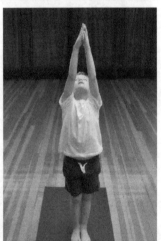
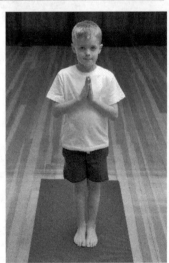

Instructions for sequence

1. Stand at front of mat.
2. Inhale reach arms up—palms together (mountain peak pose).
3. Exhale—fold body forward—fingers towards mat (rag doll with arms stretched out to mat).
4. Inhale—walk hands forward on mat come to knees (plank pose).
5. Exhale—tuck toes (down dog).
6. Inhale—look to front of mat.
7. Exhale—walk feet towards front of mat.
8. Inhale—come back to standing, reach arms up, palms together (mountain peak pose) .
9. Exhale—palms together in front of chest.
10. Repeat 2–3 times.

Breath

▷ ujjayi
▷ open mouth breath

Benefits

Strengthens cardiovascular, respiratory, digestive and circulatory systems; stretches and tones muscles in entire body; strengthens immune system; calms nervous system; energizes the brain and body; strengthens the vestibular and proprioceptive systems.

Body awareness

▷ Whole body awareness

Additional sequenced poses

Incorporate any sequence of standing poses, backbends, forward bends, inversions and twists to provide vestibular input.

TRIANGLE (TRIKONASANA)

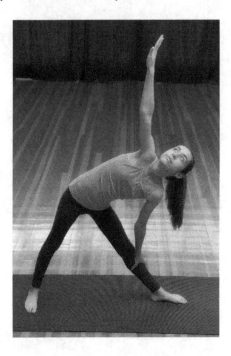

Instructions for pose

Use colored stickers or wristbands to designate right (red) and left (lavender), as described on page 40 if needed.

1. Stand sideways on mat.

2. Spread legs wide.

3. Point toes of right foot towards front of mat (child's front heel should line up with back inner arch of foot—or close).

4. Reach arms out to the side.

5. Bend to the right.

6. Bring right hand down toward mat.

7. Right hand can rest on right shin or on yoga block (avoid pressing hand on right knee).

8. Reach left hand up toward sky.

9. Look up to fingers reaching to the sky.

10. Breathe.

11. Repeat on opposite side.

Breath

▷ ujjayi

▷ open mouth

Benefits

Expands chest and shoulders; strengthens thigh muscles; increases neck and hip mobility; stretches spinal muscles, calves and hamstrings; energizes.

Body awareness

▷ feet

▷ arch

▷ heel

▷ hips

▷ arms

▷ hands

Visualization

Imagine the shape of a triangle. Turn your body into a triangle.

Modifications

Slight bend in front knee, shorten stance, gaze can be down at the mat or looking forward in front of the body.

EAGLE (GARUDASANA)

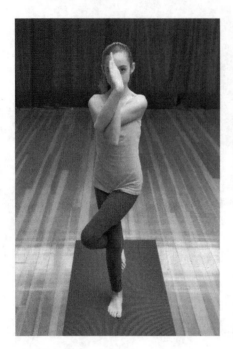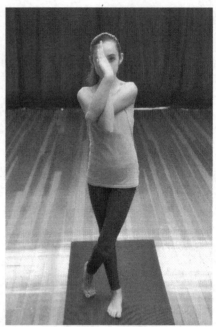

Instructions for pose

Use colored stickers or wristbands to designate right (red) and left (lavender), as described on page 40 if needed.

1. Stand tall with feet apart.
2. Reach arms forward.
3. Bring right arm under left arm.
4. Bend elbows.
5. Palms together (or close to each other).
6. Look at a spot on the wall (head facing forward).
7. Lift right leg and bend right knee.
8. Cross right leg over left leg.
9. Wrap right toes behind left leg.
10. Look forward at spot on wall.
11. Breathe.
12. If you fall out it's ok! Just come back in and try again!
13. Repeat on other side.

Breath

▷ ujjayi

Benefits

Strengthens ankles, legs, knees and hips; stretches and releases tension in shoulders and upper back; increases focus and concentration; calms the nervous system.

Body awareness

▷ feet

▷ knees

▷ legs

▷ arms

▷ elbows

Visualization

Imagine an eagle sitting high in a tree, standing strong, watching from above.

Modifications

Bring toe to mat alongside the ankle of the standing foot.

SHARK (SHALABASANA)

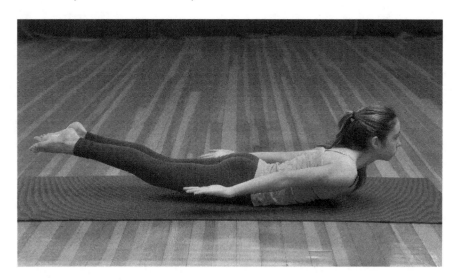

Instructions for pose

1. Lie on belly.
2. Arms to side of body (fingers pointing back towards heels).
3. Chin to mat.
4. Inhale—lift shoulders and feet off mat.
5. Reach fingers back towards heels.
6. Exhale—shoulders and feet come down.
7. Repeat 4–5 times.

Breath

▷ ujjayi
▷ open mouth breath

Benefits

Strengthens the muscles of the spine, buttocks and backs of the arms and legs; stretches the shoulders, chest, belly and thighs; improves posture; stimulates abdominal organs; supports digestion; helps relieve stress.

Body awareness

▷ belly
▷ shoulders
▷ arms
▷ fingers
▷ low back
▷ legs
▷ feet

Visualization

Imagine a shark swimming in the ocean, legs are tail and arms are fins.

Modifications

Arms reach out in front.

TREE (VRKSASANA)

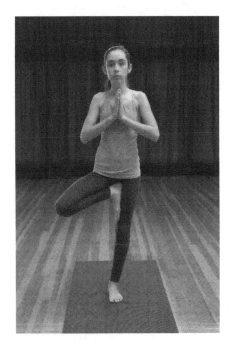 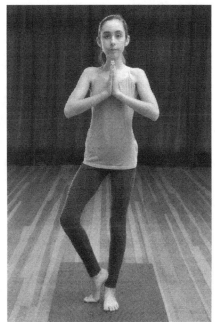

Instructions for pose

Use colored stickers or wristbands to designate right (red) and left (lavender), as described on page 40 if needed.

1. Stand on mat, feet together.

2. Bring right foot to inside of thigh or calf.

3. Find spot on wall to look at (drishti).

4. Bring palms together in front of chest.

5. Inhale.

6. Exhale—grow your branches.

7. Reach arms up to sky.

8. Breathe.

9. If you fall out, it's ok! Just come back into pose and try again!

10. Repeat on opposite side.

Breath

▷ ujjayi

▷ open mouth

Benefits

Strengthens thighs, calves, ankles and spine; stretches the groins and inner thighs, chest and shoulders; improves sense of balance and focus; increases self-esteem.

Body awareness

▷ feet

▷ knee

▷ belly

▷ arms

▷ palms

Visualization

Imagine being a tree, roots growing out through foot, arms raise up as branches (grow your branches).

Modifications

Bring heel to ankle so toes are still on the floor instead of inside of calf or thigh, keep palms together at chest instead of reaching them up. Use chair, table or wall to support balance.

AIRPLANE (DEKASANA)

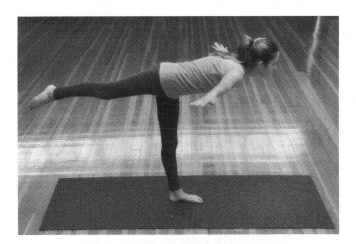

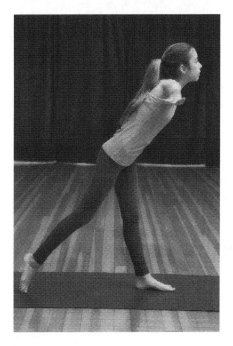

Instructions for pose

Use colored stickers or wristbands to designate right (red) and left (lavender), as described on page 40 if needed.

1. Stand in middle of mat.

2. Inhale—reach arms out wide to the side.

3. Exhale—lean front of body forward.

4. Lift right leg.

5. Stand strong on left foot.

6. Look at a spot on the ground in front of you (drishti).

7. Breathe.

8. If you fall out, it's ok! Just come back into the pose and try again!

9. Repeat on opposite side.

Breath

▷ ujjayi

▷ open mouth

Benefits

Strengthens legs; stretches arms and chest; stimulates the abdominal organs, diaphragm and heart; improves sense of balance and focus; increases self-esteem.

Body awareness

▷ toes

▷ feet

▷ legs

▷ knees

▷ arms

▷ shoulders

Visualization

Imagine being an airplane flying in the sky, arms as wings.

Modifications

Keep the top of back toes on the mat while leaning torso forward; hold a chair or table while balancing.

COBRA (BHUJANGASANA)

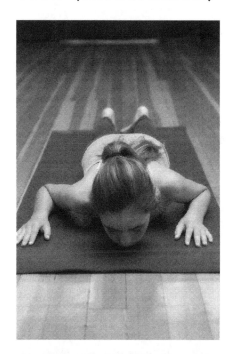
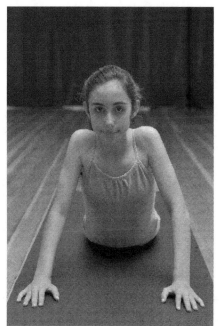
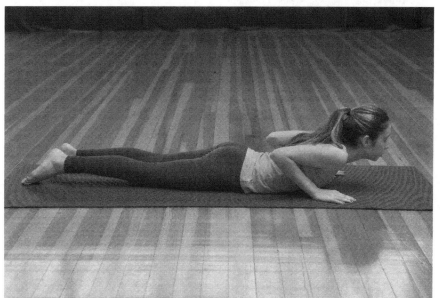

Instructions for pose

1. Lie on belly.

2. Chin on mat.

3. Bring hands under shoulders (or to outside of shoulders).

4. Palms on mat.

5. Inhale—press palms into mat, straighten arms and lift shoulders off mat.

6. Exhale—hiss like a snake, shoulders back to mat.

7. Repeat 2–3 times.

Breath

▷ ujjayi

▷ open mouth

Benefits

Strengthens the spine; stretches chest, shoulders and abdomen; supports digestion; helps relieve stress and fatigue; opens the lungs; therapeutic for asthma.

Body awareness

▷ palms

▷ elbows

▷ shoulders

▷ belly

▷ top of feet

Visualization

Imagine being a cobra snake, peeking up from the grass.

Modifications

Keep elbows bent.

STAR

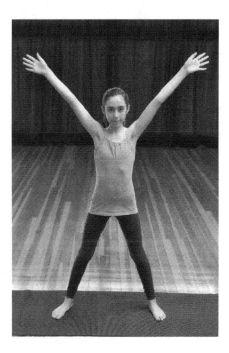

Instructions for pose

1. Stand on mat.
2. Spread legs wide to outside of mat.
3. Heels in, toes out.
4. Inhale—reach up—palms facing front of room.
5. Exhale—spread arms and fingers wide.
6. Stand tall.
7. Breathe 5–6 breaths.

Breath

▷ ujjayi
▷ open mouth

Benefits

Stretches and lengthens body in all directions; aligns spine; improves posture; energizes the body; strengthens legs, ankles, abdomen and back; improves circulation and respiration; helps relieve stress and anxiety and improve concentration and focus; supports balance; improves mood and self-esteem.

Body awareness

▷ feet

▷ heels

▷ legs

▷ belly

▷ arms

▷ hands

▷ fingers

Visualization

Imagine your body as a star with five points (head, two arms and two legs).

Modifications

Can do pose lying down on a mat.

WARRIOR 2 (VIRABHADRASANA II)

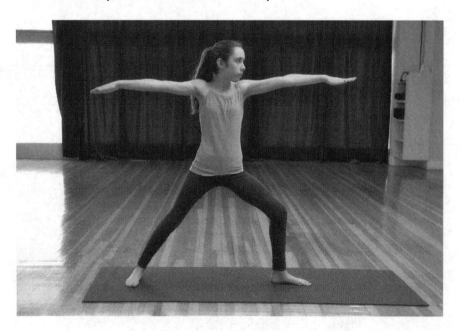

Instructions for pose

Use colored stickers or wristbands to designate right (red) and left (lavender), as described on page 40 if needed.

1. Stand sideways on mat.

2. Spread legs wide. Press hand with bent knee onto wall to stabilize.

3. Bring right foot toward front of mat (child's front heel should line up with back inner arch of foot—or close).

4. Bend right knee.

5. Stretch arms out to side.

6. Look to the right.

7. Inhale and exhale.

8. Repeat instructions for opposite side.

Breath

▷ ujjayi

▷ open mouth

Benefits

Stretches hips, groins and shoulders; improves circulation and respiration; energizes limbs; opens chest and lungs; supports digestion; improves balance and concentration; increases self-esteem.

Body awareness

▷ feet

▷ heels

▷ knees

▷ hips

▷ belly

▷ shoulders

▷ arms

▷ palms

▷ fingers

▷ neck

Visualization
Imagine being a brave warrior, standing strong and tall.

Modifications
Less bend in knee, shorten stance.

FLAMINGO

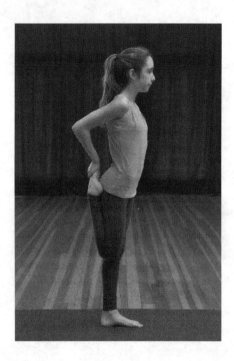

Instructions for pose
Use colored stickers or wristbands to designate right (red) and left (lavender), as described on page 40 if needed.

1. Stand on mat—feet together.
2. Find a spot on the wall to look at (drishti).
3. Bring right heel to your bottom.
4. Reach back and grab top of right foot with right hand.
5. Stand strong on left leg.

6. If you fall out, it's ok! Just come back into pose and try again!

7. Breathe.

8. Repeat on opposite side.

Breath

▷ ujjayi

▷ open mouth

Benefits

Strengthens feet, ankles and legs; increases focus and concentration; encourages balance and coordination; calms the nervous system; helps reduce anxiety; increases self-confidence and self-esteem.

Body awareness

▷ hands

▷ legs

▷ feet

▷ heel

▷ bottom

Visualization

Imagine being a pink flamingo standing on one leg.

Modifications

Use opposite arm of bent leg to support balance by bringing it wide out to the side. Hold onto chair, table or wall with free arm to support balance.

HAPPY BABY (ANANDA BALASANA)

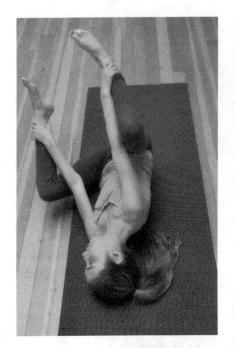 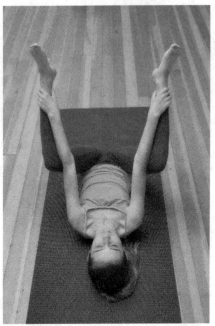

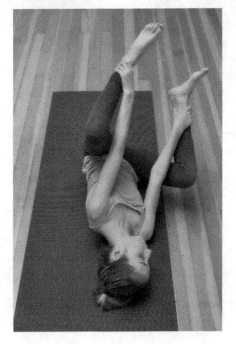

Instructions for pose

1. Lie on back.
2. Bend knees.
3. Spread knees wide.
4. Grab hold of ankles.
5. Keep back of head on mat.
6. Inhale.
7. Exhale—rock to the right.
8. Inhale—come back to center.
9. Exhale—rock to the left.
10. Repeat 3–4 times.

Breath

▷ ujjayi
▷ open mouth breath

Benefits

Stretches inner thighs and groins; relieves tension in lower back; calms brain; helps relieve stress and fatigue.

Body awareness

▷ hands
▷ back
▷ knees
▷ ankles (inner thighs and calves if modified)

Visualization

Imagine a happy baby playing with toes, rocking back and forth.

Modifications

Have child grab inside of thighs or inside of calves if needed. Have child stay in center without rocking if rocking is too difficult.

BRIDGE (SETU BANDHA SARVANGASANA)

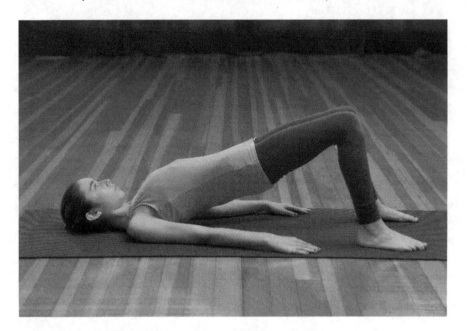

Instructions for pose

1. Lie on back.
2. Bend knees.
3. Make space in between knees (hip width).
4. Feet on floor (parallel to each other).
5. Bring arms to side, palms on floor.
6. Press palms into mat.
7. Lift hips.
8. Breathe.

Breath

▷ ujjayi

▷ open mouth breath

Benefits

Stretches chest, neck, spine and hips; strengthens back, buttocks and hamstrings; supports digestion; improves circulation; stimulates lungs and thyroid glands; helps alleviate anxiety and mild depression; reduces fatigue and insomnia; calms the nervous system; reduces backache and headache.

Body awareness

- ▷ arms
- ▷ palms
- ▷ feet
- ▷ knees
- ▷ hips

Visualization

Imagine a rounded bridge. Make your body into a rounded bridge.

Modifications

Place a yoga block lengthwise under the sacrum/lower back.

OPEN BOOK/CLOSE BOOK

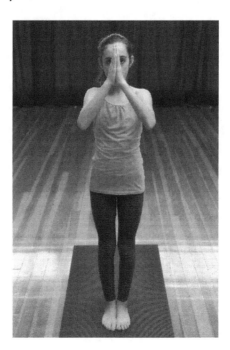

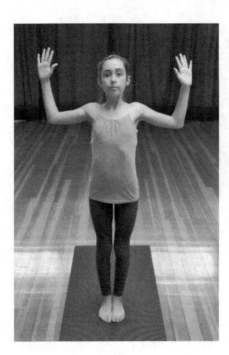 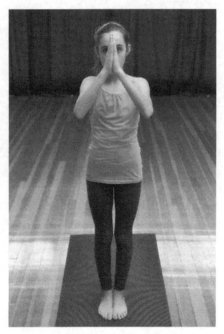

Instructions for pose

1. Stand tall on mat.

2. Bring palms together in front of forehead. Encourage child to bring their elbows together if possible.

3. Open arms.

4. Inhale—spread elbows wide. Encourage child to lift elbows to shoulder height.

5. Palms face forward.

6. Exhale—bring palms back together in front of forehead. Encourage child to bring their elbows together if possible.

7. Repeat 4–5 times.

Breath

▷ ujjayi

▷ open mouth breath

Benefits

Opens up front of body, the heart, lungs, diaphragm and chest; supports better posture; prepares the body for deeper breathing; calms and centers the mind.

Body awareness

- arms
- elbows
- palms

Visualization

Imagine opening a book and closing a book.

Modifications

This pose can be done seated in a chair.

ROLLER COASTER TWIST

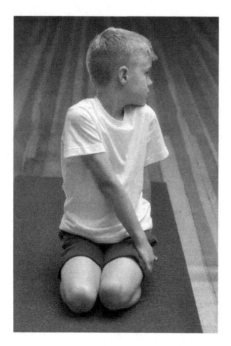 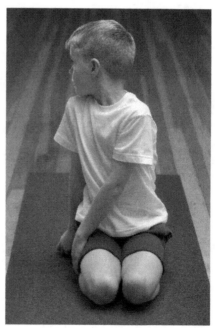

Instructions for pose

Use colored stickers or wristbands to designate right (red) and left (lavender), as described on page 40 if needed.

1. Sit back on heels.
2. Sit up tall.
3. Inhale.
4. Cross left arm over to right.
5. Exhale.
6. Twist to the right (gentle twist).
7. Bring right arm on mat behind body.
8. Look over right shoulder.
9. Breathe.
10. Repeat on opposite side.

Breath

▷ ujjayi
▷ open mouth

Benefits

Massages and cleanses internal organs; supports digestion; restores and maintains normal spine rotation; calms the nervous system.

Body awareness

▷ hips
▷ heels
▷ arms
▷ spine
▷ shoulders

Visualization

Imagine your spine twisting like roller coaster tracks.

Modifications

Have the child place their back hand on a block or book behind them.

GAMES USING ASANAS

It is important to note that yoga is not intended to be competitive. The games suggested in this chapter are to teach the child yoga poses and breathing strategies in a fun and interactive way. Although some of the games have the option to have winning players, it is not necessary to have a winner. Learning skills such as turn-taking, good sportsmanship, being a leader, interacting with others and following directions are important lessons when learning social skills and how to get along with others. It is up to the adult to know how the child will respond to friendly competition and to make modifications to the game based on knowledge of the individual child. Participants in the game can include family members, siblings, peers, friends and any other individuals that are a support to the child.

GO TAKE A POSE

This game requires at least two players.

What does the child learn?

▷ communication skills

▷ vocabulary

▷ turn-taking

▷ counting

▷ good sportsmanship

▷ how to do poses!

Materials

▷ Pairs of yoga cards with matching yoga poses or breaths (these cards can be printed photos of the child or someone else in poses or magazine/printed pictures of the animals for breaths).

▷ Visual cue (if needed): Go take a pose and do you have_____?
(adult can write "Go take a pose and do you have _____?"
on a whiteboard or piece of paper or enter the cues into the child's communication device so the child has access to the verbal scripts throughout the game).

▷ Yoga mat.

How to play the game

1. The adult passes 5–7 cards out to the child and the other player/players and places spare cards in a pile.

2. Each player checks to see if they have matching poses or breaths.

3. Players set pairs aside.

4. One player asks for example: "Do you have tree pose?"

5. If the other player has the matching pose, they give the card to asking player.

6. If the other player does not have the matching card, they say "Go take a pose."

7. The asking player does the pose then takes a card from the pile.

8. If the player gets a match from the pile, player sets pair aside.

9. Players take turns.

10. The game is over when one person has no more cards in their hand.

11. The person with no cards left in their hand is the winner!

YOGA MEMORY GAME

This game requires at least two players.

What does the child learn?

▷ communication

▷ vocabulary

▷ memory skills

▷ turn-taking

▷ counting

▷ yoga poses and breathing

▷ good sportsmanship

Materials

▷ Pairs of 8–12 matching yoga cards with matching yoga poses or breaths (these cards can be printed photos of the child or someone else in poses or magazine/printed pictures of the animals for breaths).

How to play the game

1. Lay all cards face down on a table.
2. Player chooses a card.
3. Player chooses another card.
4. If the cards don't match the player puts the cards back in their spots and the next player goes.
5. If the cards match the player puts the matching set aside and takes another turn. Player keeps going as long as player gets a match.
6. When all of the cards have been matched, players count their cards.
7. The one with the most cards is the winner!

GUESS THE POSE

This game requires at least two players.

What does the child learn?

▷ vocabulary

▷ communication

▷ turn-taking

▷ yoga poses

▷ memory

▷ good sportsmanship

Materials

▷ printed pictures of yoga poses (pictures can be of the child or someone else doing yoga poses)

▷ name of poses written on recipe cards or strips of paper or names of poses in child's augmentative communication device or iPad

▷ yoga mat

How to play the game

(This game may require an additional person to support the child in the game depending on level of independence.)

1. Lay pictures of poses out next to yoga mat for player doing pose.

2. Lay words out in space on floor or at table for the player guessing the pose.

3. Demonstrating player chooses a picture of a pose while the guessing player has eyes closed or is facing away, then demonstrating player places the picture of the pose where the guessing player won't see it.

4. Demonstrating player demonstrates the pose.

5. Guessing player tries to guess the pose (can use words on table to help with memory).

6. If the guessing player gets the pose right they keep the card. (Option to lay two cards in front of child with correct pose and choice of another pose so child can choose which pose is the correct pose to support child with memory and set the child up for success.)

7. Players take turns.

8. After all of the cards have been demonstrated, players count their cards.

9. Whoever has the most cards is the winner!

MUSICAL POSES

This game requires multiple players (at least four players).

What does the child learn?

▷ listening skills

▷ attention skills

▷ counting

▷ yoga poses

▷ good sportsmanship

Materials

▷ rubber circles (or colored pieces of cardstock to put on floor)

▷ music

How to play the game

1. Adult places rubber circles (or colored paper) to equal one fewer than total number of children (e.g., five rubber circles for six children) on floor in a circle.

2. Adult plays music as children walk around circle, stepping on rubber circles.

3. When music stops, children attempt to step on remaining circles and then children must do a yoga pose on the circle.

4. The child who did not make it on a circle sits out.

5. Adult takes another circle away.

6. Repeat until only one child is left on a circle.

7. Child left stepping on and doing yoga pose on last circle wins!

YOGI SAYS

This game requires multiple players (at least four).

What does the child learn?

▷ listening skills

▷ attention skills

▷ imitation skills

▷ leadership skills

▷ turn taking

▷ yoga poses

▷ socialization skills

▷ good sportmanship

Materials

▷ yoga mats

▷ popsicle sticks

How to play the game

1. Adult has children space their bodies or stand on mats.

2. Adult says, "Yogi says do_____ pose." (e.g., "Yogi says do airplane pose.")

3. Children do pose (adult can model pose if needed).

4. Adult tries to trick children during game by omitting Yogi and saying "Do _____ pose."

5. Children who do pose without *Yogi says* in sentence get a popsicle stick in their container.

6. Children can take turns being Yogi.

7. Game can last for as long as adult decides (use a timer to signal end of game).

8. Children count their popsicle sticks.

9. At the end of the game whoever has the *fewest* popsicle sticks is the winner!

MIRROR ME

This game requires two players.

What does the child learn?

▷ imitation skills

▷ social skills

▷ turn-taking

▷ yoga poses

▷ breathing strategies

▷ emotions

▷ perspective-taking

Materials

 ▷ star or sticker chart (the adult can reinforce the child's imitation skills by putting a sticker on a chart after mirroring pose or breath)
 ▷ adult, sibling, peer or any other person who can guide child in doing poses and breathing

How to play the game

Pose

1. Guide and child stand facing each other.
2. Guide models steps of pose one motion at a time.
3. Guide can do physical prompting if necessary.
4. Child mirrors guide.

Emotion and breath

1. Guide models facial expression such as anger.
2. Child mirrors expression.
3. Guide models volcano breath to release anger.
4. Child mirrors volcano breath.
5. Continue for as many poses and breaths as desired.
6. If child is capable, child and guide can switch so the child is the demonstrator and the guide mirrors the child.

This is a great game for practicing, recognizing and imitating body movements, facial expressions and breaths. If children are capable, pairing two children together to play mirror game can facilitate socialization and perspective-taking.

ART ACTIVITIES

The adult can engage the child in learning and doing poses by allowing them to color or draw their own images. The adult can print black and white images of animals, landscapes or objects and allow the child to create their own images to use when practicing poses. Having the images on hand while doing the poses will help activate the child's memory and imagination.

Suggested art activities:

▶ Make a sun for Waking the Sun pose.

▶ Make animals to match animal poses.

▶ Make apples and oranges for apple and orange picking.

▶ Color a beach scene for wave breath and visual imagery.

▶ Have child make color cards.

▶ Have child color and cut out an image to use on the wall for drishti.

▶ Have child draw pictures of emotions to use during breathing activities.

▶ Design a butterfly for butterfly pose.

7

SELF-REGULATION
AND BODY AWARENESS

Children with autism and other special needs may struggle with a variety of "sensory" issues or, more specifically, sensory integration dysfunction. Sensory processing or sensory integration (SI) is a term that refers to the way the brain or nervous system receives messages from the senses and then turns those messages into appropriate behavioral and motor responses. Our senses provide information about the physical state of our body and the environment around us. There is a constant flow of sensory signals coming to our brain at any given moment. When our brain is functioning or is "wired" normally, it is able to organize the vast amount of sensory input coming in, which allows us to move and behave normally. Sensory integration dysfunction is a condition in which the sensory signals or messages are disorganized, therefore mixing up and disorganizing the child's behavioral and motor responses.

Occupational therapist and neuroscientist A. Jean Ayres, PhD, likens the brain to a traffic policeman: when functioning normally the brain locates, sorts and orders sensations in a well-organized and integrated manner. She describes sensory integration dysfunction as a neurological "traffic jam" that prevents certain parts of the brain from receiving the information needed to interpret sensory information correctly (Ayers 1979). Because the brain is a processing organ, which processes sensations both from the inside of the body and from the outside environment, many aspects of a child's functioning can be affected when their brain does not integrate this information correctly. Sensory integration involves motor processing such as vestibular (balance, where our head is in relation to our body); proprioception (where our joints are in relation to each other, understanding the orientation of one's body in space) and kinesthesia (movement and orientations of one's limbs, how fast our body is moving). A child with sensory integration dysfunction may struggle with all or some of these motor skills, the difficulty being that there are three subsystems with signals coming into the brain at the same time. The brain of a child with sensory integration dysfunction lacks the ability to process these signals all at one time in order to facilitate whole brain communication.

Not only does sensory integration dysfunction affect motor processing, but it also has a significant impact on emotional and behavioral regulation. Our senses tell us how aroused or alert we should be and how to process emotions such as anger or anxiety. We make decisions about how we should be feeling emotionally and physically based on sensory information from both inside and outside of the body. This gathering and processing of information allows us to self-regulate our arousal states as well as our emotions or behavioral responses. Sensory integration dysfunction can make it difficult for a child to perform the simplest daily tasks and may also make it difficult for a child to participate in a variety of activities in the home or school setting. In many cases, children with sensory integration dysfunction can be easily distracted by the vast amount of stimulus in their environment. This factor can have a direct correlation with their ability to focus in their environment and stay engaged or attend to a task or activity. This is due to the difficulty in processing multiple stimuli or sensations in the environment or in their own body. In many cases children with sensory integration dysfunction will hyper-focus on objects, thoughts or stimuli due to their difficulty integrating more than one sensation at a time. A child's heightened response to stimuli in their environment can also cause increased anxiety as well as behavioral issues. A significant reason for the behavior issues can be that the different parts of the child's brain are not working together to allow the child to assimilate information and interpret how to respond emotionally to a sensation or stimuli.

Disorganization in a child's sensory processing affects the five senses we are familiar with, visual (sight), auditory (sound), olfactory (smell), tactile (touch) and gustatory (taste). Many children with sensory integration dysfunction may have heightened or adverse responses to bright lights or movement, loud or unexpected noises, textures of clothing, food or other objects, various smells and the taste of different foods. Due to their inability to process this sensory input of the five senses, as well as vestibular and proprioceptive sensory input in an organized manner, their responses to outside sensory stimuli can be deemed inappropriate and difficult to understand. Stanley Greenspan, joint author of *The Challenging Child*, describes it this way:

> Imagine driving a car that isn't working well. When you step on the gas the car sometimes lurches forward and sometimes doesn't respond. When you blow

the horn, it sounds blaring. The brakes sometimes slow the car, but not always. The blinkers work occasionally, the steering is erratic, and the speedometer is inaccurate. You are engaged in a constant struggle to keep the car on the road, and it is difficult to concentrate on anything else. (Greenspan and Salmon 1995, p.4)

Children with sensory integration dysfunction experience this same frustration of their system not working efficiently or cohesively. They are engaged in a constant struggle to keep all or parts of their system running.

Smith and Gouze (2004) describe sensory integration as having three complementary processes; *sensory modulation, sensory discrimination* and *motor planning*. They describe sensory modulation as the brain's ability to adjust the intensity of response to sensory stimuli. The "modulation" is the ability to respond to some sensory input while tuning out other sensations (Smith and Gouze 2004, p.39). An example would be tuning out the sound of an air conditioner or a fan while watching a television show. While this could be distracting to an individual without sensory integration dysfunction, they are more equipped to modulate their responses or set up an environment to support their specific sensory sensitivities. Children with sensory integration dysfunction often lack the ability to choose the environment to support their sensory needs as well as the ability to modulate their response to sensory stimuli. According to Smith and Gouze (2004), sensory discrimination is the ability to distinguish one sensory experience from another. When our sensory system is functioning normally, we are able to interpret and assimilate sensory stimuli from the environment and make decisions based on this information. We are able to identify whether sounds are near or far, whether they are threatening or insignificant and we are able to adjust our responses based on this ability to discriminate. Many children with sensory integration dysfunction lack this ability to discriminate, which can greatly affect their ability to organize and execute decisions in their daily lives. Smith and Gouze describe motor planning or praxis as "the ability to translate sensory input into organized, purposeful motor output" (2004, p.41). They say that "motor planning involves six factors, (1) coming up with an idea about the action, (2) having an accurate sense of where the body is, (3) starting the action, (4) executing the steps in the appropriate sequence, (5) making adjustments as needed and (6) knowing when to stop the action" (Smith and Gouze 2004, p.41). Many children with sensory integration deficits have difficulties in the area of motor planning and may struggle with one or many of the factors described above which can affect their ability to self-regulate and modify their actions or responses to internal and external stimuli.

"Self-regulation is the ability to self-organize—to control one's activity level and state of alertness as well as one's emotional, mental or physical responses to sensations" (Smith and Gouze 2004, p.240). Specific breathing activities and poses suggested in Chapters 4, 5 and 6 will support the child in learning strategies to regulate arousal states, express emotions and control emotional responses. Specific yoga poses can be taught to a child with sensory integration dysfunction or sensory processing deficits to provide appropriate vestibular and proprioceptive stimulation, to increase sustained attention and focus, to support behavioral self-regulation, to develop body awareness and to support whole brain/body communication and functioning. Yoga for children with sensory integration difficulties teaches them how to regulate their own systems, similar to tuning a radio. I explain to my students that they are in control of their own radios. If they are feeling static or not quite right they can switch to a different station or adjust the knob so the station comes in clearer. They can adjust their volume up or down, depending on their energy or arousal state. I liken the breathing strategies and poses to that of the knobs and dials on a radio. When children with sensory integration difficulties are able to tune in to their bodies and learn strategies to self-regulate on their own, they develop a sense of self-confidence and feel more in control of themselves and the world around them.

The poses and breathing activities suggested in this chapter are to support the child in regulating and balancing their sensory systems in order to self-regulate and self-organize their responses to sensory stimuli, strengthen their motor-planning skills and develop more brain/body connection. For purposes of this book and the connection to yoga and sensory integration, the parts of the sensory system that will be focused on are the "hidden" sensory systems, the vestibular system and the proprioceptive system, as well as the action of crossing the midline to balance the two hemispheres of the brain.

The vestibular and proprioceptive systems when functioning in a healthy way, work together to keep us grounded, connected to our bodies and aware of the world around us. These two systems work together to tell us where to sit in a chair so we don't fall off, how much distance to have between ourselves and others, how to move our limbs and bodies in different settings and how to regulate our posture and muscle tone. Both systems play an important role in a child's ability to self-regulate and self-organize.

VESTIBULAR SYSTEM

The vestibular system, the area of the brain that is responsible for balance, is also responsible for regulating attention, concentration and emotional/behavioral stability. Vestibular input helps us maintain our balance by telling us whether we are at rest or in motion. Vestibular input tells us the rate at which we are moving as well as registering the movement of objects around us. Children with sensory integration dysfunction may have difficulty knowing what rate to move their bodies such as when to go fast and when to slow down. They have difficulty planning and organizing their motor movements based on information from their bodies and the environment around them. They may attempt to get vestibular input by running, spinning or pacing in their environment. Although these physical movements are ways for a child with sensory integration dysfunction or sensory processing deficits to get vestibular input, they may not always be appropriate behavioral or social responses. Sequences of yoga poses that encourage the child to move from one pose to the next such as back bends, forward bends and twists provide vestibular input that help balance out the vestibular system and create a sense of calm and groundedness. Poses in which the child moves their head in many directions and positions provide vestibular input and strengthens the vestibular system.

Poses for vestibular input:

Balancing poses—Boat, Eagle, Tree, Airplane, Flamingo (see Chapter 6).

Standing poses—Triangle, Warrior 2 (see Chapter 6).

Inversion pose—Down Dog (see Chapter 7).

Forward bending poses—Rag Doll, Giraffe (see Chapter 6).

Sun salutation sequence—(see Chapter 6).

PROPRIOCEPTIVE SYSTEM

Proprioception provides input of where our bodies are in space and provides a sense of groundedness as well as a feeling of comfort and stability. Proprioception gives us the ability to coordinate the movements in our bodies. Sense receptors in our joints and muscles send signals to the brain, the brain organizes these signals and then tells our body the appropriate movement or response for coordinating movements in the body, such as placing one foot in front of the other for walking or striding, holding hands in the right position to catch a ball, bringing a fork to our mouth, holding an item with the appropriate amount of pressure, how much pressure is needed to balance on one foot, etc. Children with sensory integration dysfunction may find coordination of these day-to-day movements challenging and frustrating. Children with sensory integration dysfunction may attempt to get proprioceptive input through unusual or inappropriate behaviors such as banging into a wall or objects in a room, jumping up and down in a repetitive manner or banging their head or other parts of their bodies with their hands or fists. Stretching and compressing or deep pressure activities provide proprioceptive input. Many yoga poses include stretching, compression of the joints and deep pressure movements.

Poses for proprioceptive input:

Stretching—Puppy Pose (see Chapter 6), Down Dog (see Chapter 7).

Compression of joints—Modified Plank (see Chapter 6), Triangle (see Chapter 7).

BALANCING POSES FOR VESTIBULAR AND PROPRIOCEPTIVE INPUT

Balancing poses are thought to develop the cerebellum, the part of the brain that controls the body in motion. They may also improve memory, focus and concentration, as well as physical coordination and grace. The weight of the body shifted to just one area creates a natural compression in the joints, making these poses soothing for the proprioceptive sensory system as well.

Additional poses for Proprioceptive Input

SUPINE TWIST

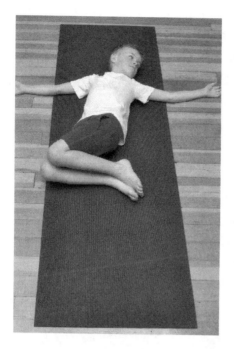 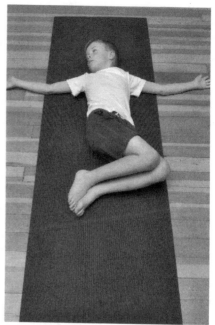

Instructions for pose

1. Lie on back.
2. Bend knees in towards belly.
3. Inhale.
4. Exhale—bring knees over to right side.
5. Stretch arms out to side.
6. Look to the left.
7. Breathe 4–5 deep breaths.
8. Inhale—knees back to center.
9. Exhale—bring knees to the left.
10. Stretch arms out to the side.
11. Look to the right.
12. Breathe 4–5 deep breaths.

Breath

▷ ujjayi

▷ open mouth breath

Benefits

Massages and cleanses internal organs; supports digestion; restores and maintains normal spine rotation; calms the nervous system.

Body awareness

▷ back

▷ knees

▷ head

▷ arms

TUG-OF-WAR

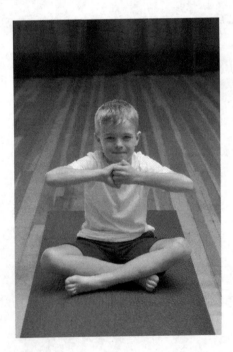

Instructions for pose

1. Sit cross-legged.

2. Bend elbows.

3. Inhale—lift elbows up.

4. Grab fingers (left palm facing body, left palm facing out).

5. Exhale—tug fingers.

6. Repeat on opposite side (right palm facing body, left palm facing out).

Breath

▷ ujjayi

▷ open mouth breath

Benefits

Increases strength in hands and fingers; helps develop fine motor skills; strengthens the vestibular system; calms the nervous system.

Visualization

Imagine playing tug-of-war with your hands.

Body awareness

▷ hands

▷ fingers

▷ arms

▷ elbows

TWISTED TRIANGLE (PARIVRTTA TRIKONASANA)

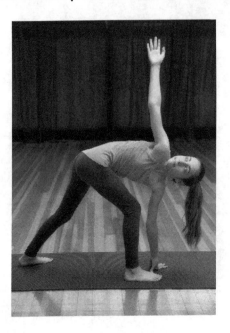

Instructions for pose

Use colored stickers or wristbands to designate right (red) and left (lavender), as described on page 40 if needed.

1. Stand sideways on mat.
2. Spread legs wide.
3. Bring right foot towards the front of mat, toes pointing forward.
4. Back foot turns in 40 degrees.
5. Heels slightly in, toes slightly out.
6. Inhale.
7. Exhale—bend sideways.
8. Reach left arm towards mat.
9. Place left hand or tips of fingers on mat (can place hand on shin).
10. Reach right arm high.
11. Look forward or up at right hand.

Breath

▷ ujjayi

▷ open mouth breath

Benefits

Strengthens and stretches legs; stretches the spine and hips; opens chest to improve breathing; supports digestion; supports balance and focus; therapeutic for asthma; strengthens proprioceptive system.

Body awareness

▷ feet

▷ heels

▷ toes

▷ hips

▷ arms

▷ hands

▷ head

▷ neck

Modifications

Bend front knee slightly, look forward toward front so neck is not twisted. Place a yoga block under bottom hand.

Deep pressure

Deep pressure can be calming, grounding and supportive to children with sensory processing issues. Poses that provide deep pressure activate the parasympathetic nervous system and can help to decrease anxiety, tension and nervous energy. These include: Rock, Sponge, Self-hug, Eagle, Down Dog, and Fetal Pose (see Chapter 6 for information and instructions). Fetal Pose varies slightly here as the child is hugging his knees into his chest for deep pressure.

ROCK

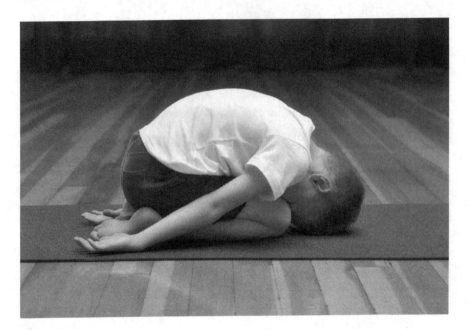

SPONGE

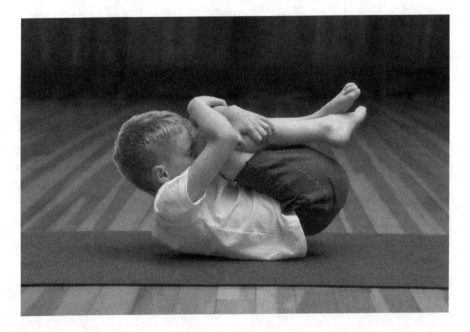

SELF-HUG

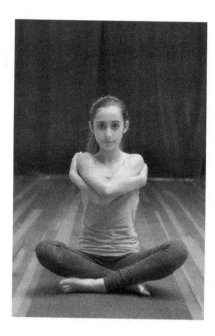

EAGLE

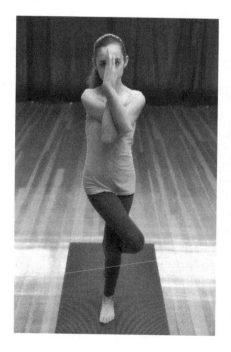 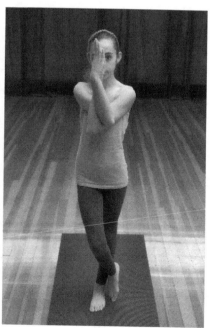

DOWN DOG

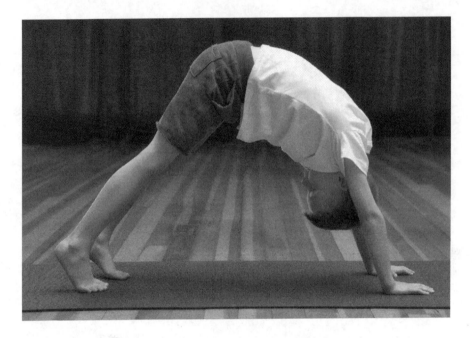

FETAL POSE

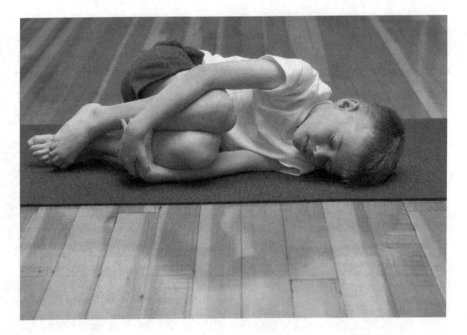

RESTING POSE (SAVASANA) WITH DEEP PRESSURE

Using a light sand bag, large pillow or several folded blankets on the chest with arms crossed or on the legs during resting pose provides deep pressure on the upper body and lower body. It is important that the sand bags are not too heavy (particularly on the chest). Be aware of the child's breathing to be sure the child can breathe with ease and comfort. Folded blankets and pillows can also be used to place on limbs (arms, legs, hands, feet) in order to create a more grounding and calming effect while the child is in savasana. Using an eye pillow during savasana may also increase relaxation.

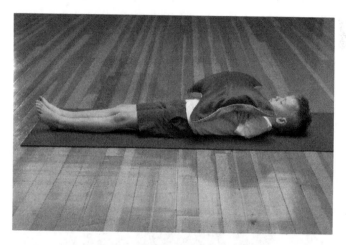

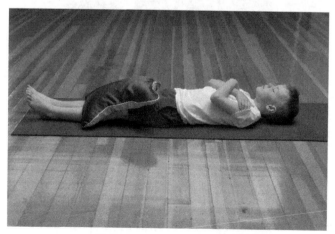

CROSSING THE MIDLINE

Another important factor in working through sensory processing disorders is doing physical activities which cross the midline. Murdoch (1987) explains how learning occurs in the entire brain but that each side of the brain prefers certain tasks and processes certain information. For instance, the left hemisphere of the brain prefers tasks such as logic, time-oriented tasks, verbal tasks and sequencing information. The right hemisphere prefers tasks such as space-oriented tasks, non-verbal tasks and images, pictures and metaphors. The action of crossing the midline, one body part from one side crossing over to the other side, forces both sides to communicate and activates the corpus callosum, the nerve fibers that join the two hemispheres of the brain. Actions that cross the midline organize the nervous system and balance the two hemispheres of the brain. Many children with sensory integration dysfunction or sensory processing deficits struggle with motor activities which require crossing the midline. It is thought that crossing the midline will support left and right brain connection and if practiced repetitively can even support the brain in developing new neuro-pathways.

Poses for crossing the midline and accessing both sides of the body:

Crossing the midline—Twisted Triangle (Utthita Trikonasana) (see page 158), Apple Picking (see Chapter 8).

Accessing both sides of the body—any poses where the pose is practiced on both the left and right side, such as Warrior 2, Triangle, Flamingo, Airplane, Eagle, Tree, Seated Twist (see Chapter 6).

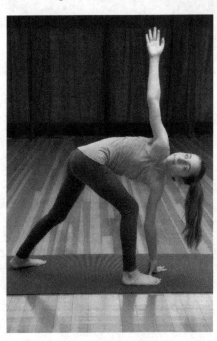

BICYCLE

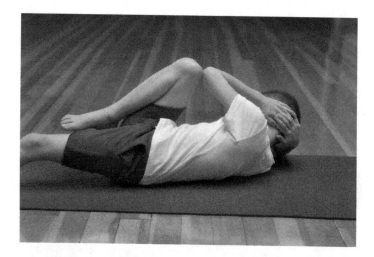

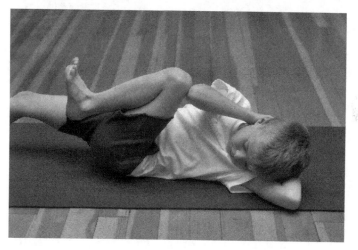

Instructions for pose

Use colored stickers or wristbands to designate right (red) and left (lavender), as described on page 40 if needed.

1. Lie on back—legs straight.
2. Clasp fingers behind neck.
3. Elbows wide.
4. Inhale—bring right knee to chest.
5. Exhale—bring left elbow to right knee.
6. Inhale—straighten right leg, shoulders to mat, bend left knee to chest.

7. Exhale—bring right elbow to left knee.

8. Repeat 3–4 times on both sides.

Child can move more slowly or go faster depending on energy level, ability and preference

Benefits

Develops core strength and flexibility; increases energy; strengthens proprioceptive system.

Body awareness

▷ elbows

▷ shoulders

▷ knees

Visualization

Imagine pedaling the pedals on a bicycle. What color is your bicycle? Do you want your bicycle to go fast or slow? Where do you want to go on your bicycle?

Modifications

Straighten arm instead of bending elbow and reach to outside of opposite leg.

EYE-TRACKING

Some children with special needs may struggle with eye-tracking weakness and visual perception, which can affect their visual processing abilities, attention to visual movements and ability to track from left to right when reading text. This eye-tracking exercise will strengthen the muscles in the eyes and enhance tracking ability. This action also crosses the midline, supporting balance of the left and right hemispheres of the brain.

SNEAKY PEEK

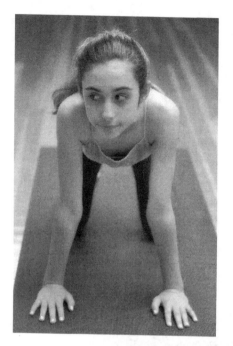

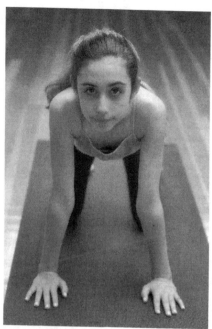

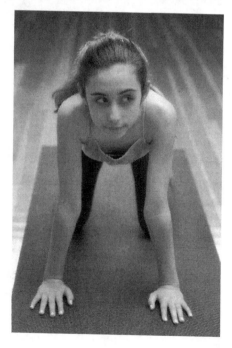

Instructions for pose

1. Pose can be done seated or on hands and knees. The child can choose to be an animal that walks on all four legs when on their hands and knees.

2. Use an object that is of interest to the child or attention grabbing.

3. Tell the child they are going to "sneak a peek" of the object with their eyes.

4. Ask the child not to move their head, only their eyes.

5. Move the object directly in front of the child.

6. Move the object to the right and tell the child to peek with their eyes.

7. Tell the child to follow the object.

8. Move the object back to center.

9. Continue to encourage the child to follow the object with their eyes only.

10. Move the object to the left.

11. Tell the child to peek with their eyes.

12. Repeat 4–5 times.

ACTIVITIES FOR ACCESSING (OR BALANCING) LEFT AND RIGHT HEMISPHERES OF THE BRAIN.

Alternate nostril breathing (See Chapter 4)—Access to left and right brain hemispheres.

Breathing in through your left nostril accesses the right "feeling" hemisphere of your brain, and breathing in through your right nostril, will access the left "thinking" hemisphere of your brain. Alternating the breath between each nostril allows access to and activates the "whole" brain.

Build muscles in eyes—track back and forth in tree pose, mountain pose, etc. Tabletop look left with eyes—look right with eyes—use a visual of something.

It is important to note that a child with special needs may not meet all of the criteria to be specifically diagnosed with sensory integration dysfunction but may display sensory processing deficits, exhibiting many of the same symptoms and challenges of sensory integration dysfunction. The suggested poses in this chapter can support any child with sensory processing difficulties or sensory integration imbalance in learning breathing strategies and poses to support them with motor planning and self-regulation.

8

CHAIR YOGA

Chair yoga can be done at home, in an office, in an airport, on a plane, in the car, in the classroom and in many other environments. Chair yoga is a great alternative for children with poor muscle tone or mobility issues where standing postures would be difficult, as well as for children in wheelchairs. Chair yoga is a great way to practice quick yoga stretches and breathing strategies with minimal preparation or disruption to the environment.

What you will need:

- a chair, couch, bench or any other space where a child can sit
- enough space for the child to move arms and upper/lower body freely
- visuals.

OPEN BOOK/CLOSE BOOK

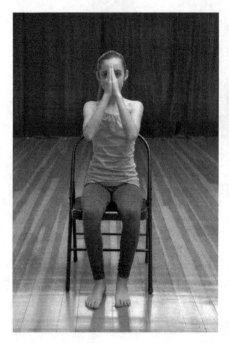 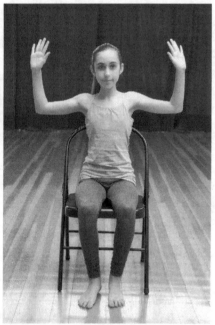

Instructions for pose

1. Sit tall in chair.
2. Palms together in front of face.
3. Inhale—open arms back with elbows bent. Encourage child to bring elbows to shoulder height.
4. Open book.
5. Exhale—palms back together in front of face.
6. Close book.
7. Repeat 4–5 times.

Breath

▷ ujjayi
▷ open mouth breath

Benefits

Opens up front of body, the heart, lungs, diaphragm and chest; supports better posture; prepares the body for deeper breathing; calms and centers the mind.

Body awareness

- palms
- elbows
- arms
- head

Visualization

Imagine a book opening and closing. Think of your favorite book.

APPLE PICKING

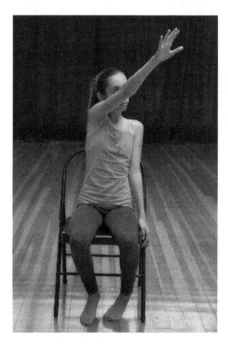 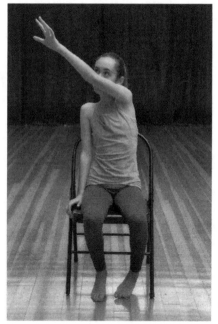

Instructions for pose

Use colored stickers or wristbands to designate right (red) and left (lavender), as described on page 40 if needed.

1. Sit up tall.

2. Inhale—reach right arm across body.

3. Pick apple, closed fist.

4. Exhale—bring arm back to side and drop apple in bucket.

5. Repeat 4-5 times.

6. Repeat on opposite side.

Breath

▷ ujjayi

▷ open mouth breath

Benefits

Crosses midline to support whole brain communication; stretches arms, shoulders and fingers; strengthens hand grip; energizes the brain; calms the mind.

Body awareness

▷ arms

▷ fingers

Visualization

Imagine reaching across to pick an apple from an apple tree. What color is the apple? How does the apple taste? Is it sweet or sour? Is it soft or crunchy? What does the apple smell like?

HEEL LIFT

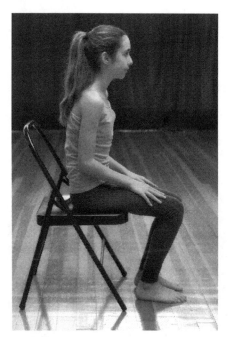 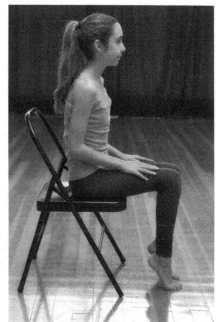

Instructions for pose

1. Sit up tall on edge of chair.

2. Feet on floor.

3. Palms down on knees.

4. Inhale—lift heels.

5. Exhale—lower heels to ground.

6. Repeat 4–5 times.

Breath

▷ ujjayi

▷ open mouth breath

Benefits

Stretches bottom of feet and ankles and toes; strengthens calves.

Body awareness

▷ toes

▷ heels

Visualization

Imagine lifting up on to toes like a ballerina.

SEATED TWIST (ROLLERCOASTER TWIST SITTING IN CHAIR)

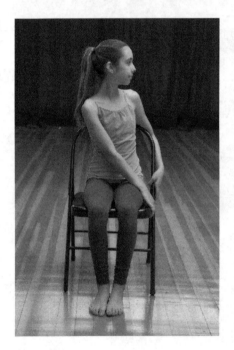 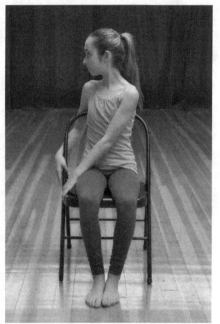

Instructions for pose

1. Sit up tall.
2. Inhale.
3. Cross right arm over to left.
4. Exhale (left arm can wrap around back of chair or come to the seat of chair behind child's bottom).

5. Twist to the left (gentle twist).

6. Look over left shoulder.

7. Stay for 2–3 breaths.

8. Repeat on opposite side.

Breath

▷ ujjayi

▷ open mouth breath

Benefits

Massages and cleanses internal organs; supports digestion; restores and maintains normal spine rotation; calms the nervous system.

Body awareness

▷ arms

▷ torso

▷ shoulders

▷ neck

▷ head

Visualization

Imagine your spine is a twisting rollercoaster track.

SHOULDER SHRUG (I DON'T KNOW, LET IT GO)

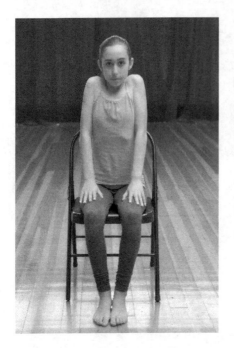 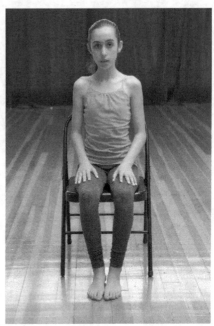

Instructions for pose

1. Sit up tall.
2. Palms down on lap.
3. Inhale—shrug shoulders up to ears ("I don't know.")
4. Exhale—relax shoulders down ("Let it go.")
5. Repeat 3–5 times.

Breath

▷ open mouth breath

Benefits

Relieves tension in shoulders and neck; relieves stress, anxiety and worry.

Body awareness

▷ shoulders

▷ hands

Visualization

Think of something that makes you worried, anxious or is frustrating to you. Use your shoulder shrugs to let it go.

SQUEEZE ORANGE JUICE

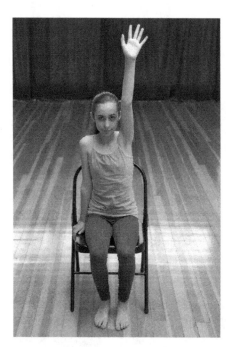 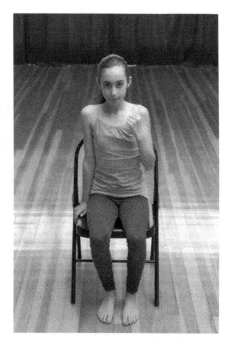

Instructions for pose

Use colored stickers or wristbands to designate right (red) and left (lavender), as described on page 40 if needed.

1. Sit up tall.
2. Inhale—reach right arm high.
3. Spread fingers wide.
4. Exhale—squeeze hand into fist.
5. Bring fist down in front of right shoulder.
6. Repeat 4–5 times.
7. Repeat on opposite side.

Breath

▷ open mouth breath

Benefits

Stretches arms, shoulders and fingers; strengthens hand grip; energizes the brain; calms the nervous system.

Body awareness

▷ arms

▷ fingers

▷ shoulders

Visualization

Imagine picking an orange from a tree and squeezing juice from the orange. How does the orange smell? How does the orange juice taste? Is it sweet or sour?

BUTTERFLY TO COCOON

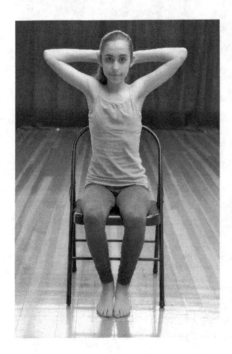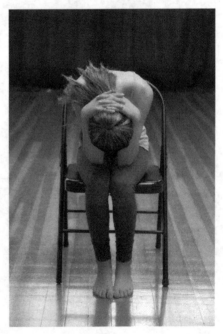

Instructions for pose

1. Sit up tall.
2. Clasp fingers behind neck.
3. Inhale—spread elbows wide.
4. Exhale—bring elbows together.
5. Bring forehead to lap.
6. Repeat 4–5 times.
7. At end of repetitions allow child to rest with forehead in lap for 1–2 minutes.

Breath

▷ ujjayi
▷ open mouth breath

Benefits

Opens the front side of the body, the heart, lungs, diaphragm and chest; stretches the spine, shoulders and neck; soothes the nervous system; relieves anxiety and stress.

Body awareness

▷ arms
▷ elbows
▷ hands
▷ fingers
▷ neck
▷ head

Visualization

Imagine a butterfly, wings opening then going back into a cocoon. Think of what color your butterfly is. Feel how quiet and calm it is in the dark, warm cocoon.

SEATED MOUNTAIN

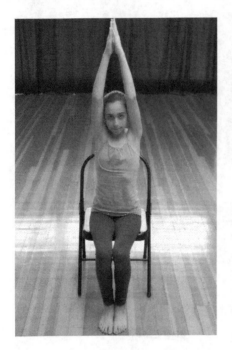 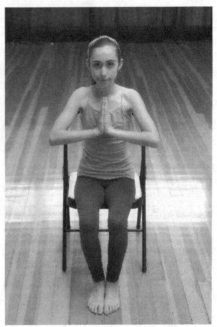

Instructions for pose

1. Sit up tall on edge of seat.
2. Palms together in front of chest.
3. Inhale—reach arms up to the sky.
4. Exhale—bring palms back together to chest.
5. Repeat 4–5 times.

Breath

▷ ujjayi

▷ open mouth breath

Benefits

Improves alignment of spine; encourages relaxation of the mind; decreases stress, anxiety and fatigue.

Body awareness

▷ arms

▷ palms

Visualization

Imagine being a strong mountain. Make a mountain peak with your hands (as child's palms come together above head).

EAGLE ARMS

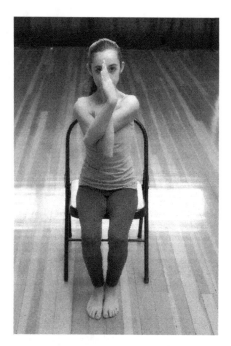 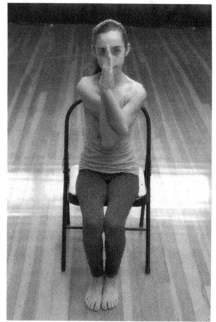

Instructions for pose

Use colored stickers or wristbands to designate right (red) and left (lavender), as described on page 40 if needed.

1. Sit up tall in chair.
2. Feet flat on floor.
3. Reach fingers forward.
4. Cross left arm over right.
5. Bend elbows.

6. Hands towards face.

7. Palms together.

8. Breathe three deep breaths.

9. Repeat on opposite side.

Breath

▷ ujjayi

▷ open mouth breath

Benefits

Stretches back muscles; releases muscle tension in neck, shoulders, chest and arms; improves circulation to upper body including heart and lungs; facilitates deeper breathing; eases stress and tension; decreases fatigue; increases energy.

Body awareness

▷ shoulders

▷ arms

▷ elbows

▷ hands

Visualization

Imagine being an eagle sitting in a tree. Hands are the beak. What color is your eagle? How do its feathers feel? What do you see from the tree?

CLOCK NECK ROLL

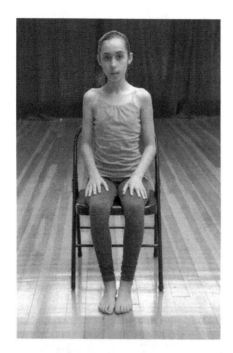
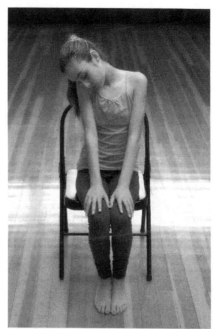
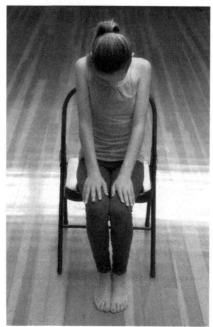
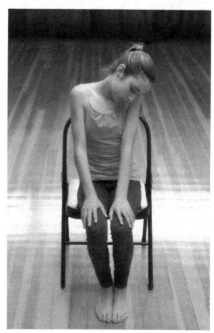

Instructions for pose

Have child do movements slowly while breathing.

Use colored stickers or wristbands to designate right (red) and left (lavender), as described on page 40 if needed.

1. Sit up tall in chair (12:00).
2. Feet on floor.
3. Inhale.
4. Exhale, right ear to right shoulder (12:15).
5. Inhale.
6. Exhale, chin to chest (12:30).
7. Inhale.
8. Exhale, left ear to left shoulder (12:45).
9. Inhale, come back to starting position.

Breath

▷ ujjayi
▷ open mouth breath

Benefits

Stretches neck and upper back muscles; relieves muscle tension in shoulders, upper back and neck; calms the mind.

Body awareness

▷ ears
▷ shoulders
▷ neck
▷ chin

Visualization

Imagine the hands of a clock moving slowly.

MIX IT UP

This can be a challenging pose for the child. There should be no pain or straining with the pose.

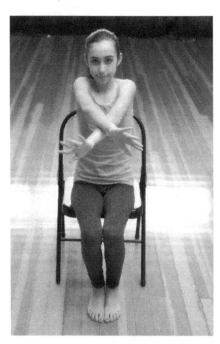 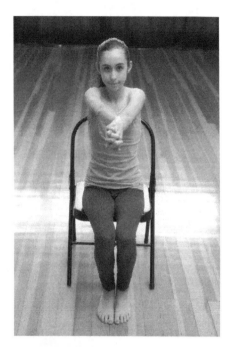

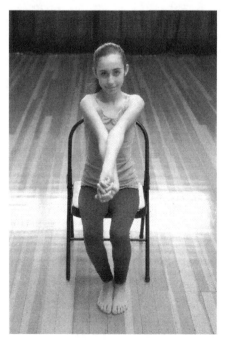

Instructions for pose

Use colored stickers or wristbands to designate right (red) and left (lavender), as described on page 40 if needed.

1. Sit tall in chair.

2. Cross right arm over left.

3. Clasp fingers together.

4. Rotate wrist so knuckles come towards chest.

5. Elbows bend.

6. Reach knuckles forward.

7. Straighten arms.

8. Repeat on opposite side.

Breath

▷ ujjayi

▷ open mouth

Benefits

Stretches wrists and arms; encourages a different movement than the body is used to and crosses the midline, which encourages whole brain communication.

Body awareness

▷ fingers

▷ wrists

▷ arms

▷ elbows

Visualization

Tell your brain to do something different with your body. Say, "Brain, let's mix it up!"

EAR STRETCH

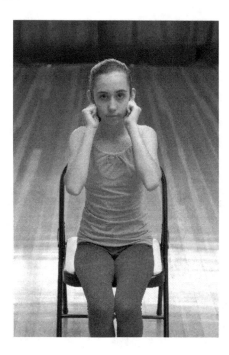

Instructions for pose

Use colored stickers or wristbands to designate right (red) and left (lavender), as described on page 40 if needed.

1. Sit up tall (can also be done lying down).
2. Grab earlobes with fingers.
3. Pull earlobes down towards shoulders.
4. Close eyes, breathe in and out.
5. Massage ears with fingers.
6. Release.
7. Repeat 3–4 times.

Breath

▷ ujjayi

Benefits

Relaxes the mind; calms nervous system; helps reduce anxiety.

Body awareness

▷ ears

▷ fingers

Visualization

Imagine stretching pizza dough. Stretch your ears like pizza dough.

REACH TO THE MOON

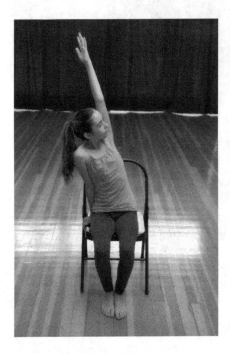 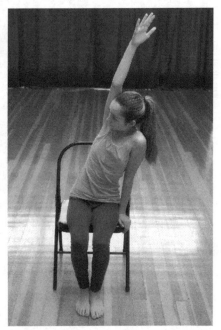

Instructions for pose

Use colored stickers or wristbands to designate right (red) and left (lavender), as described on page 40 if needed.

1. Sit up tall in chair.

2. Bring right hand down on chair next right hip.

3. Inhale.

4. Exhale—stretch left arm up and over to the right side.

5. Turn head to the left—towards left armpit.

6. Wave to the moon.

7. Breathe 2–3 breaths.

8. Inhale—sit up straight in chair (back to center).

9. Repeat on opposite side.

Breath

▷ ujjayi

Benefits

Stretches side body; increases flexibility in spine; energizes the body.

Body awareness

▷ hands

▷ arms

▷ head

Visualization

Imagine reaching fingers up to the moon.

SELF-HUG

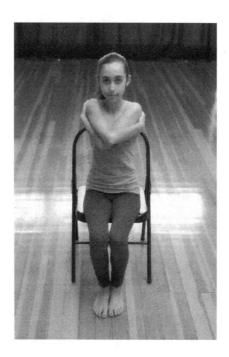

Instructions for pose

Use colored stickers or wristbands to designate right (red) and left (lavender), as described on page 40 if needed.

1. Sit up tall.
2. Reach fingers forward.
3. Cross right elbow over left.
4. Bring fingers to shoulder blades.
5. Inhale—squeeze and hug yourself tight.
6. Exhale—relax hug.
7. Repeat inhale—squeeze and exhale—relax 2–3 times.
8. Repeat on opposite side.

Breath

▷ open mouth breath

Benefits

Relieves tension in shoulders, upper back and neck; calms the mind; encourages self-love.

Body awareness

▷ fingers

▷ elbows

▷ shoulders

Visualization

When you hug your arms around yourself think of love and happy feelings.

SHOW ME TEN

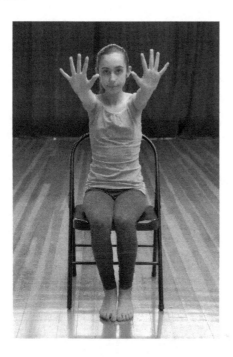

Instructions for pose

1. Sit up tall.
2. Inhale—bend elbows, reach arms back, make fists with hands.
3. Exhale—reach arms forward and spread fingers wide (showing ten fingers).
4. Repeat 4–5 times.

Breath

▷ open mouth breath

Benefits

Stretches fingers and hands; strengthens the arms; energizes.

Body awareness

▷ arms

▷ hands

▷ fingers

Visualization

Imagine you're showing the number ten with your ten fingers.

WAKE THE SPIDER

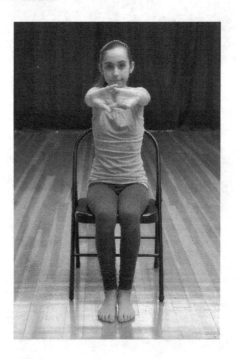

Instructions for pose

1. Sit up tall.

2. Inhale—clasp fingers together—move fingers like spider legs.

3. Exhale—stretch palms towards front of body (with fingers still clasped).

4. Breathe 4–5 breaths.

Breath

- ▷ ujjayi
- ▷ open mouth breath

Benefits

Stretches fingers, hands and wrists; energizes the limbs of upper body.

Body awareness

- ▷ fingers
- ▷ palms
- ▷ arms

Visualization

Imagine a sleepy spider moving its legs slowly, then stretching and waking up.

SUMMARY

It is my belief that children with autism and special needs have the same wants, needs and desires as everyone else. They want to be free of worry and anxiety. They want to communicate their thoughts and emotions. They want to feel comfortable in their bodies. They want to feel connected to themselves and others around them. They want to be happy and healthy. I believe the first step in helping these children to live happier, healthier lives is to teach them how to self-regulate their arousal states so they may learn to respond to stimuli in their environment more effectively. Mindful breathing, guided meditation and the practice of physical poses will support the child in responding to stressors in healthier ways. Practicing pranayama and asanas that support expression of emotions, activate the parasympathetic nervous system and bring the body and mind to a calmer state will benefit the child emotionally, physically and behaviorally. When yoga is practiced consistently, the nervous system is strengthened and has a greater capacity for enduring stress. Helping these children develop stronger nervous systems leads the way to healthier digestion, stronger immune systems, better sleep patterns, increased focus and less anxiety. Our ultimate goal after all as parents, family members and educators is to help raise calmer, happier children. Taking a holistic approach to helping these children involves looking at the bigger picture. In order to learn academics, effective communication skills, social skills and functional life skills, the child must be free of stress and tension. By minimizing the negative impact of stress on the child we are able to activate the cognitive, thinking and expressive parts of their brain. By teaching children how to self-regulate their bodies and responses to sensory input they learn lifelong coping skills. By teaching children to express their emotions and release anger, worry, fear and tension from their bodies, they learn how to self-soothe and regulate their emotions. By teaching children poses and breathing exercises, through the use of words, pictures and visualization, they develop greater language and communication skills. By teaching children body parts and connection to their own bodies through music and movement they develop a greater sense of body awareness. By teaching children how they can be in control of their emotions and their bodies' responses to stress, they develop a greater sense of self-esteem, self-confidence and self-empowerment. The physical benefits of flexibility, strength, motor skills and coordination will help children with autism and special needs navigate the world with stronger, healthier, more balanced bodies. My ultimate desire is to empower children with autism and special needs with tools that will support them throughout their life.

References

American Psychiatric Association (2013) *Desk Reference to the Diagnostic Criteria from DSM-5*. Washington DC: American Psychiatric Publishing.

Ayers, A. J. (1979) *Sensory Integration and the Child*. Los Angeles, CA: Western Psychological Services.

Bell, N. (2007) *Visualizing and Verbalizing for Language Comprehension and Thinking*. 2nd Ed. Avila Beach, CA: Gander Publishing.

Biblioteca Pleyades "The Human Brain." www.bibliotecapleyades.net/ciencia/ciencia_brain01.htm accessed on 14 November 2014.

Ehleringer, J. (2010) "Yoga therapy in practice. Yoga for children on the autism spectrum." *International Journal of Yoga Therapy 20*, 131–139.

Flisek, L. (2001) "Teaching yoga to young school children." *Positive Health 70*, 50–54.

Galantino, M., Galbavy, R. and Quinn, L. (2008) "Therapeutic effects of yoga for children: A systematic review of the literature." *Pediatric Physical Therapy 20*, 1, 66–80.

Gardner, H. (1991) *How Children Think and How Schools Should Teach*. New York, NY: Basic Books.

Genetics Home Reference (GHR) (2014) *Your Guide to Understanding Genetic Conditions: Prader-Willi syndrome*. U.S. National Library of Medicine. Available at http://ghr.nlm.nih.gov/condition/prader-willi-syndrome, accessed on July 15, 2014.

Grandin, T. (1995) *Thinking in Pictures and Other Reports from My Life with Autism*. New York, NY: Doubleday.

Greenspan, S. and Salmon, J. (1995) *The Challenging Child: Understanding, Raising and Enjoying the Five "Difficult" Types of Children*. Boston, MA: Addison-Wesley.

Harper, J. C. (2010) "Teaching yoga in urban elementary schools." *International Journal of Yoga Therapy 1*, 1, 99–109.

Iyengar, B. K. S. (2008) *B.K.S. Iyengar Yoga. The Path to Holistic Health*. London: DK Publishing.

Jensen, P. S. and Kenny, D. T. (2004) "The effects of yoga on the attention and behavior of boys with attention-deficit/hyperactivity disorder (ADHD)." *Journal of Attention Disorders 7*, 4, 205–16.

Kaley-Isley, L.,Wamboldt, M., McDunn, C. and Fury, M. (2009) "Eight week manualized yoga intervention for adolescents with anxiety, depression and medical illness." *International Journal of Yoga Therapy 19*, 1, 37–54.

Kim, J. A., Szatmari, P., Bryson S. E., Steiner D. L. and Wilson, F. J. (2000) "The prevalence of anxiety and mood problems among children with autism and asperger syndrome." *Autism Journal 4*, 2, 117–132.

Murdoch, M. (1987) *Spinning Inward: Using Guided Imagery with Children for Learning, Creativity & Relaxation.* Boston, MA: Shambhala Publications.

NDSS (National Down Syndrome Society) (2014) "What is Down Syndrome?" Available at www.ndss.org/Down-Syndrome/What-Is-Down-Syndrome, accessed on October 2, 2014.

NICHD (2006) "Disorders commonly associated or sharing features with Fragile X." Eunice Kennedy Shriver National Institute of Child Health and Human Development. Available at www.nichd.nih.gov/publications/pubs/fragileX/Pages/sub12.aspx, accessed on July 14, 2014.

NICHD (2012) "What are the symptoms of Fragile X syndrome?" Eunice Kennedy Shriver National Institute of Child Health and Human Development. Available at www.nichd.nih.gov/health/topics/fragilex/conditioninfo/Pages/commonsymptoms.aspx, accessed on July 14, 2014.

NICHD (2013) "What are the symptoms of autism spectrum disorder (ASD)?" Eunice Kennedy Shriver National Institute of Child Health and Human Development. Available at www.nichd.nih.gov/health/topics/autism/conditioninfo/Pages/symptoms.aspx, accessed on July 14, 2014.

Rama, S., Balentine, R. and Hymes, A. (2011) *Science of Breath: A Practical Guide.* Honesdale, PA: Himalayan International Institute of Yoga Science and Philosophy of the USA.

Shorter, S. M., Reinhardt, K. M., Cope, S. and Khalsa S. B. S. (2008) "The effects of Kripalu yoga on anxiety, mood and positive psychological states in adolescent musicians." *International Journal of Yoga Therapy 19*, 1, 37–54.

Smith, K. A. and Gouze, K. R. (2004) *The Sensory-Sensitive Child: Practical Solutions for Out-of-Bounds Behavior.* New York, NY: HaperCollins.

Streeter, C. C., Jensen, J. E., Perlmutter, M. R., Cabral, J. H. *et al.* (2007) "Yoga asana sessions increase brain GABA levels: A pilot study." *Journal of Alternative and Complementary Medicine 13*, 4, 419–426.

Index